The Cranial Release Technique
How CRT is Transforming Lives
by Optimizing Brain Function

William Doreste, DC
Patrick K. Porter, Ph.D.
Bob Hoffman, DC

Foreword by
Paul Drouin, M.D.

Would you like to have Dr. William Doreste, Dr. Hoffman or Dr. Porter provide a keynote, lecture or workshop on brain wellness strategies for your organization's next event? Simply call or email using the contact information provided here:

William Doreste, DC / The Cranial Release Technique, Inc.
24-38 83 St., East Elmhurst, BY 11370
917-400-1911
http://theultimatewellnesspractice.com

Patrick K. Porter PhD/PorterVision/Self-Mastery Technology
1822-6 South Glenburnie Road, #362
New Bern, NC 28562, 302-721-6677
302-721-6677 patrick@portervision.com

Bob Hoffman DC / The Masters Circle
PO Box 576, Jericho, NY 11753
516-822-5500/ bob@themasterscircle.com

Disclaimer: This book is designed to provide information in regard to the subject matter covered. It is sold with the understanding that the publisher and author are not engaged in rendering psychological advice and that the processes in this book are non-diagnostic and non-psychological. If psychological or other expert assistance is required, the services of a competent professional should be sought. The purpose of this book is to educate and entertain. Neither Awaken the Genius Foundation Co., the author, or any dealer or distributor shall be liable to the purchaser or any other person or entity with respect to any liability, loss, or damage caused or alleged to be caused directly or indirectly by this book. If you do not wish to be bound by the above, you may return this book for a full refund.

ISBN: 978-1-937111-29-8

Printed in the United States of America
10 9 8 7 6 5 4 3 2

TABLE OF CONTENTS

\#\#\#

"In today's environment, treating the body without treating the brain is like slapping a fresh coat of paint on a condemned house; it may look like improvement from the outside, but the foundation is destined to crumble."

- Patrick K. Porter, Ph.D.

Meet Your Authors

Dr. William C. Doreste, DC
Author, CEO, The Cranial Release Technique

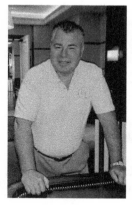

The institute is dedicated to the advancement of the Cranial Release Technique® (CRT) as a vital tool for healthcare practitioners worldwide in promoting wellness and reducing stress in patients and clients.

The Cranial Release Technique, Inc. training institute has accredited healthcare providers located in the US, Canada, Mexico, UK, Australia, Spain, South Korea, Curacao and Israel. We have also collaborated with numerous professional associations in the fields of chiropractic and other alternative medicine associations. Dr. Doreste is a 1985 graduate of New York Chiropractic College and a member the New York Chiropractic Council.

In addition to his extensive experience training practitioners in cranial-related systems, Dr. Doreste has conducted educational programs on workforce health and safety for a wide range of corporations and labor organizations. Among them are Federal Express, United Parcel Service, American Airlines, Marriott Hotels, Coca-Cola, Budweiser, New York City Emergency Medical Services, the District Council of Carpenters, and the International Brotherhood of Electrical Workers.

Dr. Bob Hoffman, DC
Author, President and CEO, The Masters Circle

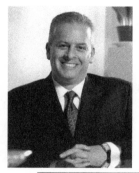

Dr. Bob Hoffman is the President of The Masters Circle, a unique Practice Building organization that has revolutionized the traditional model of coaching for chiropractors. Throughout his career, he has achieved a wide variety of honors including becoming the 12th President of the

International Chiropractors Association, Chairman of the Board of the New York Chiropractic Council, Bestselling author, sought after coach and international speaker. His reputation precedes him, as he has successfully guided thousands of chiropractors and their teams to professional excellence and personal mastery.

Dr. Patrick K. Porter, PhD

Author, President and CEO, PorterVision, LLC

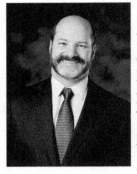

Patrick K. Porter, PhD has been on the cutting edge of brain training technology for 25 years. He was a co-developer of the MC2, the first personal light & sound brain training machine, voted "Best New Gadget of the Year" at the 1989 Consumer Electronics Show. His newest brain-training device, the MindFit Neuro-Trainer™ works to activate the brain's neuroplasticity. He is a licensed trainer of NLP and is the head of mind-based studies at the International Quantum University of Integrative Medicine (IQUIM). He is the author of six books including his newest release, Thrive In Overdrive, How to navigate Your Overloaded Lifestyle and the bestseller, Awaken the Genius, Mind Technology for the 21st Century, which was awarded "Best How-To Book of 1994" by the North American Book Dealers Exchange. He and Dr. Hoffman previously co-authored Your Flourishing Brain, a chiropractor's guide to Brain-Based Wellness..

Mind-Based Medicine for Health Care

Fifty years ago, quantum physics emerged as a new scientific standard and model for understanding reality, revolutionizing our society on many levels, sparking discussion of science vs. spirituality/consciousness, and transforming the core of our society. In the field of medicine, mind-based medicine has emerged as a major player in the application of this new perspective of reality.

When neuroscience began agreeing that brain neuroplasticity is possible, the next step was to implement technologies that allow for re-wiring the brain. This new concept has completely revolutionized the field of psychology and medicine. The old paradigm described brain neurocircuity as a fixed entity that cannot be influenced, an extension of the belief that most diseases are pre-determined by your genetics and that, fatalistically, there is nothing you can do about it.

In an updated curriculum of medicine, the new biology is redefined and expanded to include the stunning concept that your system of beliefs can actually modify your genes (Bruce Lipton, Biology of Belief, Quantum University). According to Dr. Joe Dispenza, another pioneer in this field, you can also create new behaviors by deliberately rewiring your brain (Brain & Neuroplasticity, Quantum University).Dr. Amit Goswami also points us in the direction of the possibility of creating new brain circuitry by implementing new behaviors. This subject is certainly the core of what he described as the stage of manifestation in the process of spontaneous healing (Quantum Doctor, Quantum University).

Is not the main challenge that any doctor or health practitioner encounters in his practice, "How can I support my client in creating new habits and ways of thinking, when their old habits and ways of thinking were part of the process that created the problems in the first place?" Specialized tools are required to help create the leap of awareness necessary for the client/patient to embark on the path of restoring health to an optimal level.

Dr. Patrick Porter, author and inventor of MindFit technologies, has been a major pioneer during the last decade in the field of mind-based medicine. Awaken Your Flourishing Brain, written in collaboration with Bob Hoffman, DC, is another significant contribution in this new model in neuroscience.

As a medical doctor and an educator, I was so impressed by the originality Dr. Porter's creative mind and his brain technology that I invited him to join the faculty of Quantum University in 2007 to offer the core knowledge regarding mind-based medicine to our students. Since then he has become the co-creator of our master's degree program in mind-based medicine, and he also teaches neuro-linguistic programming (NLP) and hypnotherapy at Quantum University.

Dr. Porter has made another significant contribution by making available the application of the concept of neuroplasticity in designing audio files, in conjunction with his ZenFramesTM/MindFit technology, for a multitude of problems associated with stress or psychosomatic and behavioral conditions that a doctor must deal with in daily practice. His technology can be implemented not only in medicine but also in the field of education. The main problems encountered in online education, and probably any model of higher learning, is how to facilitate and support the student in the challenging process of acquiring new information. An important factor in the high dropout rate is directly related to both a lack of motivation and to complaints of difficulty in absorbing and remembering new information often encountered by students over the age of 40. The dramatic amount of energy and money that must be invested in the mainstream model of education is certainly not worthwhile, considering that all the statics converge to declare that we are currently creating a new generation of students who find themselves jobless and in debt.

Quantum University has integrated Dr. Porter's technology to address and overcome these problems by implementing the original concept of a superlearning technology – "Quantum Superlearning Technology" – which is available to support students in America and worldwide. This system incorporates the knowledge that a whole-brain state and alpha/theta brainwave frequencies create the optimum learning environment, and that when learning occurs at the level of quantum consciousness, the information is more easily retained and recalled as needed. Dr. Porter's recorded voice, in conjunction with other aspects of the MindFit technology, guides a student through the highlights of each main course subject. These recordings can be loaded onto the student's iPad, along with other bonus relaxing and uplifting meditations and visualizations from Dr. Porter's library. "Quantum Superlearning Technology" has helped thousands of students overcome their fears and optimize their ability to focus, learn, and succeed in achieving their academic goals.

Finally, I'd like to say that Dr. Porter's contributions have been not only to offer new technology applicable to health and to the challenges of supporting new behaviors by rewiring the brain, but also to optimize the process of learning, allowing students not only to study about new concepts of potentiality, but also enabling them to achieve their own maximum potential and enhance their own well- being as they go through the learning process.

Awaken Your Flourishing Brain presents new information regarding neuroplasticity in a refreshing language available not only to students but to anybody interested in taking advantage of this strategic information in their daily lives to improve their well-being and health. Concrete solutions to the healthcare crisis can be provided by making this unique technology, supported by the latest insights in neuroscience, available to anyone interested in generating a preventive environment for their own health.

Health care is in urgent need of applications derived from a new model of understanding based on the premises of quantum physics and the new concept of neuroplasticity, applications that are affordable and easily integrated both in clinics and at home. Self-Mastery Technology (SMT), discussed previously as ZenFramesTM/MindFit technology and elaborated more fully in Dr. Porter's book, will provide individuals the power to generate health and increase their infinite potential.

Let's be realistic: new ideas are great, but without technology that reflects this new possibility of rewiring the brain, improving behaviors, and increasing health in the general population, we will not be able to make a significant difference in health care.

Awaken Your Flourishing Brain is certainly a very readable book containing critical information that should be shared with everyone who would like improve their health.

Paul Drouin, M.D.
President & Founder of Quantum University
Author of Creative Integrative Medicine

INTRODUCTION

They say anyone can do anything once they set their mind to it. They also say that there is no one standing in our way but ourselves when it comes to achieving the goals we initially set out to accomplish. These statements may sound cliché, but can anyone really deny their validity?

The thing is, you DO have the ability to change the world just by thinking that you can. No need to feel self-conscious if you believe this age-old saying. That doesn't make you an egomaniac. In fact, it defines who you are and it's that very fact that can alter the way you perceive the world around you.

Yes, that's right! You have the ability to change the world around you just by changing your thoughts—and you do that by changing how you use your brain. The best part is that it doesn't have to cost you a penny to do it and it's actually quite easy to accomplish. Read on to find out how.

What outcome do we want for you?

Our goal for you is for you to finish our journey together with a greater understanding of the 3-pound universe that inhabits the space between your ears, with the know-how for exercising and activating that most powerful computer on earth, so you can have the joyful, flourishing life that is your birthright.

We wrote this book because we know that the world cannot change until we learn how to change our own lives. As you read through these pages, we see you experiencing an awakening; we see you discovering how, by using more of your brainpower, you can change your life far more easily than you ever dreamed possible.

We see you living a life of awe and wonder as you realize that your mind need only see an image of what you truly want for you to have it, and that your brain is what we call a "servo-mechanism," which means it's always striving to prove you right.

We also see you experiencing the true joy that comes when you fall in love with yourself, your life and the world in which you live, when you discover the limitlessness of an infinite universe—including the boundless potential within your human brain.

Additionally, we see you and your family expressing far greater levels of health and vitality. We want to show you how to eliminate, reduce or remove the interference to the innate wisdom that resides within you so that the power that made your body can heal your body and keep you well. This book is about giving you the power to have more control over your brain and nervous system so you can live the life of your dreams.

Don't worry; it's easier than you think. Solutions to your every problem are available to you right now. In fact, those solutions have always been there, waiting for you to wake up and break free from the limitations you learned during childhood, to let go of the narrow mental attitude that you absorbed from the people around you, and release the stress and confusion that kept you mired in longing, despair, and the illusion of lack. We want you to realize how, when you see what you want and truly believe you can have it, the unseen forces of your mind will go about proving you right, creating a way for you to solve any problem, overcome any obstacle, and get anything and everything you want out of life.

CHAPTER ONE

The Cranial Release Technique

Chapter One - Cranial Release Technique

Dr. William Doreste is a 1985 graduate of the New York Chiropractic College and is a member of the International Chiropractic Pediatric Association and the new York Chiropractic Counsel. He is the chief executive officer of Cranial Release Technique, Incorporated, a national training institute founded in 2005. The Institute is dedicated to the advancement of the Cranial Release Technique developed by Dr. Doreste and is worldwide in promoting wellness and reducing stress. The Institute is an accredited health care provider located in the United States, Canada, Mexico, the UK, Australia and Israel.

Dr. Doreste began practice in Flushing, Queens in 1985. After practicing for more than a decade he began to realize something was missing in his practice and he began to research chiropractic and its methods. He discovered what was missing wasn't located in the spine as many chiropractors believe. He believed what was missing was in the cranium. As he continued his research he found that chiropractic has many cranial techniques but they were complicated and time consuming, sometimes taking 45 minutes or more; and they didn't resonate with what he was trying to accomplish.

Dr. Doreste learned through his research that the bones of the head move in a rhythmic pattern throughout life and this movement is responsible for the proper function of the nervous system and for optimal health. When the skull is distorted and this movement is disturbed, our health suffers and pain or illness is the result. By learning to properly manipulate the bones of the cranium, natural movement is restored, and a return to good health follows.

What emerged from his years of research was the Cranial Release Technique. This technique is a simple and powerful one that can change the physiology of the entire body in a minute or less. Dr. Doreste explains it as, "the express train to releasing restrictions, releasing physiological imbalances in the body--all through the head."

This technique is based on the anatomy and physiology of the cranial structure. By contacting the left and right sides of the head at specific anatomical points with specific amounts of force or pressure, Dr. Doreste's Cranial Release Technique gets all 22 cranial bones moving and breathing again and activates the primary respiratory mechanism.

The Cranial Release Technique, or CRT, is a hands-on approach to releasing the body's capacity to heal and regenerate itself. It can be applied in minutes but has profound effects on health and healing. This technique arose out of a new school of thought that considers the cranium and all the tissues affected by the cranium and nervous system within the approach. The entire cranium is restored to normal function with one process and the release of the bones of the skull initiates a release of all the tissues and structures associated with the cranium including the spine and pelvis, shoulders, hips, knees, the protective covering of the brain and spinal cord, the fascia and the cerebrospinal fluid. The global release of all these tissues by the Cranial Release Technique has positive effects on overall body functioning and is accomplished in minutes.

Fueled by a desire to help as many people as possible, Dr. Doreste has made it his mission to share this technique with as many alternative health practitioners as possible through his training seminars. He started sharing his technique at chiropractic conventions as well as with the Florida State Massage Therapy Association and in a few short years over 400 trained practitioners across the country are now utilizing his technique. He's also been endorsed by such chiropractors as Dr. Wayne Dyer and Dr. Dick Versendaal, DC, DCRC, DACBN.

Dr. Doreste feels that his Cranial Release Technique fits in with alternative healing modalities such as massage because when Cranial Release is performed properly the entire body relaxes. The soft tissue relaxes and the body becomes much more receptive to the therapy being performed whether it's massage or a chiropractic adjustment. And because it's such a gentle technique, it does not cause wear and tear on the body of the practitioner over time the way massage or chiropractic can. Therefore, the client gets better treatment from the practitioner and the practitioner benefits as well.

One of the most important things that the Cranial Release

Technique can do is combat the effects of stress on our bodies by restoring and enhancing wellness. We live in stressful times. Stress is physical, chemical and emotional. There is no escaping at least one of these contributors on a daily basis. It's part of being alive. When we're under this constant chronic stress, the brain hemispheres become unbalanced. Chronic stress produces a host of challenges to normal body function. The nervous system goes into overdrive and produces harmful chemicals. One hemisphere is going to become overactive and when that happens, one side of the musculoskeletal system will be tightened and over contracted. That can affect posture, the way you walk, the way you drive, the way you perform all your activities of daily living. Cranial Release counteracts the toll stress is taking on your body and brings your body back into balance.

This technique can assist with anything from aches and pains to digestive issues to the endocrine system to skin related issues. Dr. Doreste's goal with CRT is to help you with the overall function of your body. It brings the body back to homeostasis so the body can restore and heal itself efficiently and effectively. Our bodies were born to be healthy and Cranial Release helps our bodies do what they were meant to do naturally by removing any interference in the system.

Many people can be helped using Cranial Release Technique. When the body is returned to normal functioning it becomes possible for healing and repair to begin. Chronic issues can respond well to this technique, even when conventional methods have failed.

Investigation into the Cranial Release Technique and its benefits have shown that CRT has a positive effect on clients by reversing stress in the body. Most people report feeling more relaxed and at ease following a CRT session. A sense of balance and peace is noted. You have a choice in how you go about your day. Your body can either be in a protection and survival mode or a mode of health and peace. CRT can help facilitate a return to healing, repair and regeneration, which makes it an ideal part of an overall wellness program.

CHAPTER TWO

Your Evolving Brain

Chapter Two - Your Evolving Brain

We know through evolution that brain development only came about when living creatures started to move. Motor activity was the impetus to developing a brain and nervous system. Once you start to move in a purposeful way, you have to make a decision. You need to be moving towards something or away from it. Right off the bat there are choices and options. There is a split in the nervous system. One part of the nervous system will drive us towards something. The other will drive us away. From the first creature that was able to move, there was a split in the nervous system and the brain.

Everyone in the field of mind technology understands that movement is what created the brain originally and it is what creates the brain in every single human being. We're all born with primitive reflexes that allow us to interact with our world from the moment we're born. In fact, we're all born with just 25 percent of our full brain capacity. As we start to move and interact with the world and input information into our brains, we get feedback from our senses, which stimulates gene production, causing our brain cells to grow. By the time we reach age three, we have around 90 percent of our brain capacity. This massive growth is all due to our movement and interaction with the world around us.

We start to see problems in brain development in children according to the symmetry of a child's motor system at an early age. If a child has problems with suckling or breastfeeding, low muscle tone, or hasn't mastered rolling over by three to five months for example, we know there is an asymmetry in the motor system. Since they don't have a fully developed brain yet and we know the motor system is what drives the sensory system and ultimately drives the development of the brain, then we know right away there is an imbalance developing in the brain as well.

Further, we know both sides of the brain develop at different stages. The right side of the brain begins to develop more in the first two to three years, followed by the left side of the brain. If an imbalance in development is not caught and corrected early on, it leads to an imbalance in the way the brain develops. This will lead to awkward movement, poor coordination, low muscle tone--ultimately leading to subluxation or an imbalance in the alignment and function of the spine.

According to Dr. Robert Melillo, author of *Autism—The Scientific Truth About Preventing, Diagnosing and Treating Autism Spectrum Disorders-and What Parents Can Do Now,* imbalances in the spine lead to an imbalance in the feedback to the brain, ultimately altering the activity and the development of the brain. If this imbalance in the brain is too great, then the right and left side can't coordinate properly. They can't share information and you end up with what we call a "functional disconnection." This disconnection between the two sides of the brain is the leading theory as to the causes of autism, ADHD, OCD, Tourette's and schizophrenia.

What is Brain-Based Wellness?

What is Brain-Based Wellness and why is it important? This is the fundamental question that will form the foundation for this book. It will serve to provide you with the core information surrounding this topic and help you recognize the information you already know, what you need to know and how to implement what you learn into your life.

You may find yourself asking what has Brain-Based Wellness got to do with me? How is this supposed to help me? The fundamental core of any successful life is to remove the interference between the creator and the created and let the power that made the body heal the body.

Increasingly, however, we are realizing there is more to healing the body than merely dealing with physical symptoms. In fact, symptoms are the last thing that shows up in the disease process and the first thing to go away in the healing process. Trying to manage or evaluate your health based on symptoms or the lack of symptoms is both misleading and dangerous.

It is misleading and dangerous because we all know people that "felt good" and either died from a heart attack or suddenly found out that they had cancer. It is essential for us to take a different and better view of our health so that we become proactive and take deliberate actions to consciously improve our health.

Making commitments to regular exercise, eating a more natural and healthier diet, taking the necessary and appropriate supplements, meditating, getting massage, going for regular chiropractic care or using technology to help balance brain function are just some of the options available to all of us. It is important to realize that when the brain and body are brought into balance, great things can and do happen.

You can go to a doctor, but when you leave the office you're still carrying around the stresses of life, which today are greater than ever, and which caused most of your symptoms without you even knowing it. For more information on this topic, read *Thrive in Overdrive: How to Navigate your Overloaded Lifestyle, by Dr. Patrick Porter.*

Why Do We Need Brain-Based Wellness?

A recent report suggested that for most North Americans over the age of 50, their number one fear is not whether they will have enough money to see them comfortably through retirement. It's not even whether they will live a long and healthy life. The number one fear for people over the age of 50 is losing mental capacity.

Sadly, cerebral decline for many is becoming more and more a reality with instances of Alzheimer's and dementia on the rise. In fact, recently there was a major report suggesting that by the end of 2015 the number of people diagnosed with this debilitating disease would rise by 400 percent. The rise in cases of Alzheimer's and dementia in our aging population have a direct correlation to our society's continually rising stress levels and the high levels of adrenaline and epinephrine that this causes in our brains.

Continuous and excessive exposure to these hormones can interfere with our normal neurotransmitter activity. Neurotransmitters are chemicals that transmit signals from a neuron to a target cell across a synapse. They are responsible for making us feel good. When neurotransmitters are not working properly, however, as in the case of people who are continually stressed, we end up feeling down, which leads to depression. This is why people can often suffer from depression without having any outward reason to do so. This type of depression is caused by a lack of certain neurotransmitters, such as serotonin, and other necessary chemicals in the brain that help keep us balanced.

Attention Deficit Hyperactivity Disorder

In today's society, everyone has heard of ADD and ADHD. In fact, most of us know at least one person who has been diagnosed with this condition. It's interesting to note, however, that before 1975 there was no such diagnosis. We have to take this into account when we examine the statistics for ADHD. One thing we do know is that ADHD has been continually on the rise with the increase in technology. The rate of parent-reported ADHD in children between the ages of 14-17 years of age was at 22 percent between 2003 and 2007, which was an increase of 42 percent from previous reporting.

Part of this increase has to be attributed to the fact that today's society is so much more fast paced. Children are learning to do things in short bursts instead of sitting down and learning from books the way we did when we were in school. Today children can just as easily watch a TV show or a movie and learn everything they need to know without ever opening a book.

In 2007 there were approximately 5.4 million children that had received a diagnosis of ADHD, nearly 10 percent of school-aged children. That figure continues to increase. Of those diagnosed children, 2.7 million are taking medications for this condition, which is an alarming statistic. As with any drug, drugs to treat ADHD have a myriad of side effects. For example, of all the shootings that have taken place in a school setting, children who were on psychotropic medications committed 100 percent of these terrible events.

Clearly, better health through better chemistry is a paradigm and a belief that isn't working and that has failed us. It has left people seeking better and more natural solutions to their problems. It is time for us to shift our focus and intent to better health through better living and that is exactly what this book is all about.

Conditioned Hyper-Eating

The former commissioner of the FDA, who once led the government's attack on addictive cigarettes, recently published research suggesting that millions of Americans suffer from a condition called "conditioned hyper-eating." This condition is a willpower sapping drive to eat--especially foods that are high fat, high sugar and salt laden--even when they're not hungry. This condition occurs in the brain where these foods light up the brain's dopamine (pleasure sensing) pathway; the same pathway that conditions people to alcohol or drugs. The research suggests that the food industry is largely at fault for manipulating ingredients to stimulate our appetites, setting in motion a cycle of desire and consumption that has ended with a nation of overeaters who must now "retrain their brains to resist the lure."

While these findings certainly help us understand why diets fail, they do nothing to correct the ingrained eating habits that caused the weight problem in the first place. If the problem started in the brain, then we must change the brain to get lasting solutions. The Brain-Based Wellness technology that we're describing in this book is proven to naturally stimulate the brain's pleasure-sensing pathways, thus derailing conditioned hyper-eating. That's one of the reasons our weight loss programs have been so successful. Our clients can learn to easily lose weight and keep it off because we retrain the brain to change its relationship with food mentally as well as physically.

Other Devastating Effects of Stress

Besides the conditions noted previously, chronic stress can lead to high blood pressure, and undue strain on the heart. Our body's natural response to stress is to trigger a rapid release of glucose and fatty acids into the bloodstream. This is how your body can respond with strength and stamina during emergency situations. The added glucose, however, if unused by the body, can cause elevated or erratic blood sugar levels. These blood sugar swings can make you feel fatigued and can lead to diabetes. The stress-related release of cortisol can also cause a buildup of cholesterol in the arteries.

During periods of high stress, cortisol and epinephrine course through the body and signal non-essential functions to stop or slow down so that all systems essential to dealing with an emergency receive an extra boost. The immune system, which is not essential for urgent activity, temporarily stops or slows down during these peak stress periods. This system works fine when stress is short term, but when stress hormones are continually pouring into the body, the immune system suffers making you vulnerable to infection and diseases such as cancer.

Osteoporosis is a big concern for most women once they reach a certain age. We've all heard that you need plenty of calcium in your diet to help prevent osteoporosis, but what most people don't realize is that the best way to guard against osteoporosis is to keep the body in harmony. Keeping blood pressure regulated helps balance the levels of cortisol in the body, which allows the body to maintain bone density.

Another physical problem caused by high levels of stress is muscle wasting. Due to the fast pace of our daily lives, many people find it difficult to exercise on a regular basis. Loss of muscle tone is the first sign of aging, but we have more control than ever thought possible to slow down, minimize or stop this process with proper exercise. They don't understand that you need muscle to regulate your metabolism. Excess stress does not just cause mental health problems, but quite obviously physical ones as well.

Many people reading this book are probably carrying a little extra weight around the midsection. You might think it's no big deal, just a few extra pounds. You'd be wrong. Having that extra weight around the middle signifies you have insulin resistance, meaning that your cortisol levels are increasing slowly over time--and you just read about the havoc that can cause in your body.

Of course, there are lots of self-help brain training techniques out there. But the reality is that most of these games or techniques typically work on cognition using old technologies and techniques, such as rote memorization. Using Brain-Based Wellness, we can dramatically enhance the results of this brain training by building on those techniques with neurosensory algorithms designed to balance and enhance your brain function. We'll explain more about these algorithms later, but we want to make it clear that these algorithms go beyond mere words. They encompass sensation and feeling.

This is another aspect that makes Brain-Based Wellness perfectly aligned to give you the results you're looking for. When you work with this technology, you're not only getting outstanding results, you're getting an experience, and it's the experience that makes the biggest difference. By shifting your breathing, physiology and focus, we help you achieve a peak state. In this state you see immediate results and feel well cared for.

Stress Risk #1: The Heart

Whenever the fight-or-flight response is triggered, whether through real or imagined stress, an increase in heart rate, blood pressure, and breathing delivers more oxygen faster throughout the body. At the same time, a rapid release of glucose and fatty acids into the bloodstream occurs. This is how your body can respond with strength and stamina during an emergency.

Chronic stress, however, can lead to high blood pressure and undue strain on the heart. The added glucose, if unused by the body, can cause elevated or erratic blood sugar levels. These blood sugar swings can make you feel fatigued and can lead to diabetes. Stress also prompts the body to release cortisol, which can cause a buildup of cholesterol in the arteries. The bottom line: Stress can contribute to cardiovascular disease.

Stress Risk #2: The Brain

Are you one of those people who work best on deadlines? Do you use stress as a motivator? If so, you may be doing long-term harm to your brain that could cause early memory loss or may even lead to Alzheimer's disease.

You may thrive on stress because of the short-term brain boost of glucose your brain gets when you're under the gun. When this happens, your senses are heightened and your memory improves. Problems start when stress lasts more than two hours. That's when the body assumes you need more physical strength than brainpower and starts sending the glucose back to the muscles, leaving your brain short of glucose. At the same time, stress hormones impair neuron functioning. Another part of the brain, the hippocampus, associated with learning and memory, can get smaller over time due to the loss of glucose and damage to neurons. Researchers don't know the full effect of a shrinking hippocampus, but they do know that it can make you forgetful and muddle your thinking.

Stress Risk #3: The Immune System

Whenever the fight-or-flight response is triggered, stress hormones course through your body and signal the non-essential functions to stop or slow down so that all systems essential to dealing with an emergency receive an extra boost of energy. Your immune system is not required for urgent activity. Therefore, it temporarily stops or slows down during peak stress periods. This system works out fine when the stress is short term, but when the stress hormones keep pouring in, your immune system suffers, making you vulnerable to infection.

Stress Risk #4: Body Fat

Many people struggling to lose weight will ask, "Why is it that my friends can gobble up everything in sight and not gain a pound, while I nibble on salads and the scale won't budge?"

The answer lies in a powerful hormone called cortisol. Cortisol's job is to signal the body to relax and refuel after periods of stress; it's the body's way of slowing us down so that we don't burn out. Invariably, those who complain about starving themselves and still struggling to lose weight live with at least one high-stress factor that was likely causing high cortisol levels. Cortisol's message to slow down tends to make us feel tired, lethargic, and hungry. Therefore, while under the powerful influence of cortisol, our tendency is to want to lie around, watch television, and snack, thus the term, stress-eater, and the reason stress can be more fattening than chocolate. And, considering that dieting ranks 7th on the list of top ten stressors, is it any surprise they are struggling?

Cortisol also triggers fat storage in the adipose tissue of the abdomen. When the majority of weight is in the abdomen it gives one an apple appearance. More importantly, it can lead to Cushing's Syndrome, which involves storage of fat on the inside of the abdominal cavity. Cushing's Syndrome can be dangerous and may lead to diabetes and heart disease.

CHAPTER
THREE

Brain-Based Wellness
and the 21st Century

Chapter Three - Brain-Based Wellness and the 21st Century

This all sounds scary, doesn't it? How can you rid yourself of this horrifying state of mind we call stress? You can't grasp it because it's not a tangible thing. You can't handle it correctly if you have no idea of what you're supposed to do. The worst thing is there really are no beneficial drugs that you can take that will eradicate the problem in an instant either. There are no drugs that can correct a lifestyle challenge. It's a destructive chain of events that make you feel as if the whole world is against you. In other words, it's actually created out of the reactions you express when life doesn't go as you planned.

The most dangerous and hidden epidemic of the 21st Century is without a doubt the neurological epidemic, which manifests itself more and more in disorders such as Parkinson's, Alzheimer's, Epilepsy, Autism, Migraines, Depression, Chronic Fatigue Syndrome, Irritable Bowel Syndrome, Lupus, Multiple Sclerosis, Anxiety, Insomnia and the list goes on and on.

When we first opened our practices years ago, diseases such as Alzheimer's, Autism and Chronic Fatigue were almost unheard of. They were rare diseases. Today serious neurological conditions such as these, where the brain is out of balance, are reaching almost epidemic proportions. As we've already discussed, this is a result of the fast-paced, high-tech, high-stress lifestyle that we live today.

Don't shake your head and think you're safe from this malady. Stress will affect you at one time or another in your life. Once stress grabs onto anyone, it digs its debilitating claws deep into your psyche and tears down every defense you can put up. The thoughts and actions that you exert are directly proportional to the amount of stress you accumulate. It happens through us, not to us, which is what makes it very hard to control.

When we're under stress, our bodies are pumping out adrenaline and cortisol and trapping us in what we already referred to as the

Sympathetic Survival Syndrome, which is a defense psychology. This is an important term that we will review next.

Sympathetic Survival Syndrome

Your Autonomic Nervous System is a part of your nervous system that regulates key involuntary functions in the body, including heart, digestion, breathing and blood flow. This system is divided into two branches: the sympathetic system and the parasympathetic system.

To help you understand what these two parts of the nervous system do, and to keep it simple, think of their function this way: The sympathetics are for survival and the parasympathetics are for healing.

When we're trapped in a sympathetic mode, we're stuck in a fight-or-flight response, which is our innate mechanism designed to protect us from injury or attack. The problem with this response is that when we're stuck on high alert there is no room for exploration, consciousness or contribution. All our abilities are focused on our survival.

Cortisol is considered the most powerful hormone in the human body. This is because cortisol's job is survival. It can override the signals of every other hormone. When daily doses of cortisol become excessive, such as in the case of an overstressed lifestyle, Sympathetic Survival Syndrome develops and its effects are dangerous and debilitating. The effects range from anxiety, obesity and depression to heart disease, dementia and cancer.

Cortisol is a master hormone. One of its functions is to tell the body to stop tapping into fat, which our brain needs to function. Our brain is, in fact, 70 percent fat. It uses the fat stores from our body for energy. If there are high levels of cortisol in the brain it functions as a barrier, stopping the brain from tapping into the body's fat reserves. This means the brain has to cannibalize itself in order to function. This leads to shrinking of the brain, which causes some of the diseases we've already discussed such as Alzheimer's.

Another side effect of pervasive and chronic stress is adrenal exhaustion, which is in direct correlation to the constant production and over-production of epinephrine (adrenaline) in the brain. Adrenal exhaustion can have very serious consequences; one of which is sleep disturbance. Whether you have trouble falling asleep or staying asleep, insomnia is another epidemic that is sweeping through our population--affecting more than 40 million people in the United States alone.

Sleep disorders can be not only distressing to the individuals suffering from them, but they can also be dangerous, causing such things as low blood sugar, constant fatigue, low immune function, anxiety and depression. These things can lead to the abuse of alcohol, food or drugs to cope with the symptoms. Sadly, the tragic effects of stress don't end there.

Another common side effect of adrenal exhaustion is chronic fatigue and low energy, which also has been rising at alarming rates.

The emergence of Sympathetic Survival Syndrome and Brain-Based Wellness is of extreme importance. Stress and the diseases it causes are reaching epidemic proportions in our modern world--and it's only going to get worse. If you were to take an honest evaluation of your life, you'd find that the majority of the time you are stressed out and suffering from the disorders and diseases related to that stress. We are all stressed at work, at home, culturally stressed, time stressed, money stressed, activity stressed and relationship stressed.

Once the Sympathetic Survival Syndrome is activated, the sympathetic system is continually revved up with little or no time for recovery, which leads to problems on every level. This creates an amazing opportunity for you to really make a change in your life and create the life you've always wanted.

Let's take a moment to review over what we've learned about Sympathetic Survival Syndrome: All forms of stress stimulate your sympathetic nervous system and cause sympathetic and parasympathetic imbalance. When stress is ongoing, it creates a neurological cascade of events that leads to Sympathetic Survival Syndrome. When we're stuck in this survival mode, our ability to heal, grow, love, and flourish is greatly diminished. The brain and nervous system are both compromised. Today the number of people trapped in sympathetic survival mode is reaching epidemic proportions. People are constantly in fight-or-flight with no recovery time. We must learn how to unwind, rebalance and heal ourselves.

When our brains become imbalanced (sympathetic overload), unfortunately, our body always follows and becomes imbalanced as well. We call this sickness and disease. How that sickness or diseases shows up is different in each and every person depending on where their "weak link" is. This imbalance can show up as eczema or migraines or allergies or back pain or as high blood pressure depending on the weakness in each individual.

Why is Stress Such a Problem Today?

The reality is we can't escape the lifestyle of the 21st century. We have to learn new mechanisms for dealing with the stresses of life to prevent them from causing problems for us, both physically and psychologically. If you're reading this book, you no doubt already have some awareness of what a Brain-Based Wellness approach can do for you.

You may be wondering what's so different about stress today compared to 50, 20 or even ten years ago? Stress is something that has had a constant presence throughout the ages. The stress response is something that's been evolving over thousands of years, created originally as a survival technique.

The problems associated with stress are becoming so prevalent in today's society, because we're constantly bombarded with it from the technology that was designed to make our lives easier. We are constantly exposed to electromagnetic frequencies from cell phones and electronics. We encounter colorings, dyes, preservatives, pollution, traffic--all are causing stress. We have money worries, family and career worries, global uncertainty and a new pressure to perform at higher levels than ever before in history.

Even modern entertainment has a negative effect. Rather than sitting out in nature fishing or spending time with our families as our ancestors did, we plant ourselves in front of 60-inch television sets watching shows depicting terrifying events, violence or non-stop action. We also add booming surround sound systems to make it all the more real. Your brain doesn't know the difference between real or imagined, so it reacts to these stressful images as if they were happening to you.

Let's be clear about this: stress causing the sympathetic fight-or-flight mechanism is not a bad thing, however, it must be balanced with the relaxation response from your parasympathetic nervous system for you to be healthy. It is the chronic, constant, never-ending fight/flight without any relaxation response that is the cause of all disease physically and mentally.

This really is a new generational problem. In the past we only saw this type of stress reaction in people who were exposed to extreme stress, such as a soldier in a combat zone. Today more and more people's daily lives are bombarded by stress, like someone who is in a combat zone. Daily they are barraged by too much information, expectancies and experiences. People want to find a wellness solution, a drug-free solution, and a doctor-supervised solution to their stress problems. People who are incorporating the use of regular and specific chiropractic care and the Mindfit System with Self-Mastery Technology audio sessions are finding just that solution.

We believe that Brain-Based Wellness is the solution. Based on the statistics in the last chapter, the majority of the population would benefit from a mind/brain-based wellness program--the solution to our society's stress problem. You may find yourself a little skeptical of these claims, but we can assure you, we're not just saying we have the answer. We have the science, experience and statistics to prove that we have the answer.

For sure, we cannot remove or eliminate the stress in your life; but we can erase, minimize and neutralize it in your brain and nervous system before it does damage.

We conducted our very first study in Arizona in the 1980s when we came out with the first portable light and sound machine. We put our device in 30 chiropractic offices to conduct a study on the efficacy of our device on school-aged children and grades.

All the participants in the study were of school age and had an average grade of B or lower. We found that within three months of using light and sound technology, the average grades had gone up by at least one grade point. B students became A students. C students became B students.

Need more proof? Many leading universities are researching the efficacy of Brain-Based Wellness. Stanford University holds a symposium every year about this subject. The term they use is brain-wave entrainment. They are recognizing the importance of the problem in society today and the need to address it. They are investigating primarily how to get people's brain wave patterns back into balance and are achieving phenomenal results.

Moscow State University is another leading research facility in the area of brain-computer interfaces. In fact, Dr. Alexander Kaplan, who designed the brain wave training algorithms that we use in our MindFit unit, is also the head of the Human Brain Research Group at the university and also heads the government project on stress diagnoses in elementary and university students.

In this chapter we're going to present a number of different strategies relating to brain wellness. The Brain-Based Wellness concept has been in development since the 1980s and it's time has now come.

We are living in the most stressful time in human history. Our world is fast-paced and high-tech. The average number of times someone picks up their Smartphone is 150 times a day; and if you've ever observed someone who thought that they lost their Smartphone, you would see what a stress response really looks like. We are constantly bombarded with stress. We are barraged with more stress than we consciously realize, with things such as electromagnetic frequencies affecting our brains and nervous systems without our awareness.

You should be aware that electromagnetic frequencies or EMFs are everywhere. Between cell phones, televisions, microwaves, blow dryers, computers, fluorescent lights and airplanes to name just a few, we're being bombarded with different electromagnetic frequencies all the time, all of which have a negative and detrimental effect on your brain and nervous system.

These EMF waves are damaging our natural brain waves and neurological patterns. They have a harmful effect on our health and the scariest thing is the ordinary person on the street is completely unaware that it's happening, because EMFs can't be seen, tasted, or measured in our day-to-day lives. It's important that we are aware of the negative effect EMFs have on our brains and our bodies.

Several people have conducted studies about the long-term effects of using cell phones and the detrimental consequences that it can have on your health, but the majority of these studies have been conducted with the view to investigating whether cell phone use causes cancer. Little is known about the other effects that cell phone use can have on our brains and our brain wave states. For example, taking a brain scan while a patient uses a cell phone shows that the radiation emanating from the cell phone penetrates into your brain and goes all the way through to the other side.

What's more important for people to know is that radiation does not dissipate as soon as you finish your phone call. It stays in your brain for prolonged periods of time. It was also found that after phone use, brain wave patterns are found to be abnormal and continue to be abnormal for an extended period of time, which stresses the brain.

An example of this is the study conducted by Ivan Pavlov with his dogs. In this experiment, Pavlov used a bell as a natural stimulus. Whenever he gave food to his dogs, a stimulus that caused salivation, he also rang the bell. After repeating this procedure numerous times he tried ringing the bell without presenting food. Surprisingly, the bell on its own caused an increase in the dogs' salivation.

The dogs learned an association between the bell and the food causing a new behavior. Because this response was learned or conditioned, it is called a conditioned response. The neutral stimulus, the bell, had become a conditioned stimulus.

Our brains and bodies react just like Pavlov's dogs. They become conditioned over time. For example, every time we use our cell phones the abnormal brain wave patterns are triggered and soon start to form a pattern. Before you know it, those altered brain waves are occurring even when we aren't using our cell phones. This alteration to our brain waves can lead to a lack of concentration, memory loss, inability to learn and aggressive behavior.

A study released at the 2013 annual meeting of the American Society of Hypertension in San Francisco found that talking on a cell phone causes systolic pressure to rise significantly. Systolic pressure is the higher number in a blood pressure reading and is the one that doctors are concerned with as a risk factor for cardiovascular disease. Additionally, cell phone use has been shown to consistently spike your Beta brain wave activity, adding significant stress to an already overtaxed brain.

Children's brains aren't patterned yet, so they are more susceptible to the re-patterning, which usually occurs naturally through our life experiences, but that is now being altered by the excessive use of cell phones and other technologies. This is why it's so important to learn how to re-train the brain back into its natural state.

Physical stress, chemical stress and emotional stress all translate into brain stress. When the brain is stressed, it goes out of balance; and as we learned in the previous chapter, when the brain is out of balance the body always follows. This is what creates sickness and disease in the body. The good news is as we reboot, re-harmonize and normalize the brain, the body follows and starts to heal, repair and regenerate back to normalcy.

People in our society today are stressed past capacity and are in what's called sympathetic overload. They are stuck in Sympathetic Survival Syndrome. Brain-based wellness produces astounding results in combating this syndrome. It's the most powerful and effective antidote to stress we've come across in 35 years and there is no better way to create balance, symmetry, harmony, healing and health in the body.

It is interesting to note that every major medical textbook states that the brain and nervous system are the master control systems regulating and controlling every other system in the body.

Some of the greatest researchers and scientific minds in the world have been focusing on this essential issue of brain-based wellness. How can we re-pattern and re-balance the brain? The research being conducted in universities around the world right now is aimed at helping us live longer lives and age gracefully. Everyone wants to have intact memory and maintain concentration. We not only want to have a body that can function well into old age, but sharp minds as well.

Brain-Based Solutions

What are some brain-based solutions that can help the body deal with stress? The first thing that can help is deep breathing exercises. You must change your breathing. You must oxygenate the brain and can do so easily by breathing in through your nose deeply and out through your mouth from the diaphragm. You should be exhaling twice as long as you inhale because inhalation stimulates the sympathetic system and exhalation stimulates the parasympathetic system. First we're calming down and oxygenating the brain while putting ourselves into a more relaxed state.

Other simple things we can do that can help release stress and engage the relaxation response are taking a nice relaxing walk and being in nature. We have often asked hundreds of seminar participants to close their eyes and focus on somewhere that they can go to for relaxation. Afterwards, they share their favorite relaxation place. Some share the golf course, some are skiing down the slopes, others are at the beach, and for others it may be hiking on a scenic trail. Notice that all are outdoors, in nature and require movement.

Simple but important activities like frequent belly laughter, strong social connections and having an attitude of gratitude all neutralize our stress and stimulate our relaxation response. This need to be practiced consciously far more often if we are serious about living a longer, happier and healthier life. We'll discuss more stress-reducing techniques and methods later in the book such as meditation, yoga, proper sleep, regular chiropractic care and more.

In brain science it's a well-known fact that when the body is under stress, part of the brain literally shuts down. One of the two sides of the brain, either the right or the left, will cease to function properly when under stress. To test this theory, stand up and balance on one foot. Do a circle in the air with the raised foot. Once you've got your balance and rhythm going, use a finger to write your name in the air. The goal is to continue making circles with your foot while writing your name at the same time.

Chances are, you were not able to do both at the same time. If you couldn't spell your name because you were doing the circles, that means your right brain is dominant and your creative side is more in control. If you found you could write your name but your leg started to kick out instead of going circular, you're probably more left-brain dominant.

If one side of your brain is more dominant, this tells us that you need to train your two brains to work together. That's what our product, the MindFit, is designed to do. You can also do things such as martial arts, play an instrument or practice yoga. These activities are all whole-brain activities. People tend to use one side of their brain more than the other. The side that needs to be worked on is the dormant side. This is important work because when you're under stress--as we are on a daily basis--one side of your brain is shutting down. If you can learn to train it to stay active, balanced and working properly, imagine how much better you would be able to think, act and respond in stressful situations when clear thinking is needed the most.

People have every right to feel however they want to feel, but our job is to educate and help you understand that feeling lousy and stressed all the time is not normal and not necessary. If you don't change your belief system or retrain your brain to work at peak performance, nothing in your life is going to change. Without brain balance you'll keep doing the same things you've been doing and getting the same results you've been getting.

If you've been exposed to too much stress for too long, it's vital that you shake things up by doing the right type of brain training. This is what we specialize in with our MindFit. There is a big difference between napping and having a session of brainwave entrainment. When you fall asleep you're not changing anything. When you start to challenge the brain through what we call strategic mind-messaging, you start to change old beliefs and patterns and liberate your mind.

One of the most important things we teach people is to learn how to put themselves in a peak state. You're either in a peak state or a weak state at all times. We've all experienced peak states for short spans of time. It comes and goes and seems to be out of our control. Most of us spend the majority of our time in a weak state where your words don't come out right, your actions don't work and you feel like you're walking on eggshells.

The truth is, we're all capable of being in a peak state whenever we want or need to be. There are things we can do intentionally to get into a peak state even without brainwave entrainment technology. The first we've already covered. It's so important to breathe deeply and with intention; remembering to exhale twice as long as we inhale.

The second thing we have to do to be in a peak state is to change our physiology. Change your posture and/or how you move. No one would deny that standing is a more powerful position than sitting. Sitting up is a more powerful position than slumping or lying down. When we move with intention and confidence, we feel more powerful. A change in physiology stimulates proprioception (the ability to sense stimuli arising within the body regarding position, motion, and equilibrium) and brain function.

The third thing we have to do to put ourselves in a peak state is to focus clearly on what we want. That is the most difficult step for some people. Most people aren't even able to articulate what it is they want. They are very aware of what they don't want but when it comes to expressing wants and goals and desires they're at a loss. To be at a peak performance we need to learn to focus on the desired outcome, whatever it may be.

We also have the ability to use and practice Brain-Based Wellness to learn to automatically override anxiety and stress, training the body to go into a relaxation response and to reverse the effects of the fight-or-flight syndrome.

Stress reduction is where the technology of the PorterVision MindFit (which we'll explain in more detail as we go) really focuses. When your brain waves are out of balance, you are operating in high Beta and not able to get into the Alpha and Theta brain wave patterns needed to generate relaxation and creativity. (There will be more on brain wave patterns and how they work later on in this book.) When you can't get in sync, then the body is out of balance from the brain to the physical body or from the physical body back to the brain. Our goal is to get you to think differently about what's happening in your life and engage the methods that work to reverse the stress-effect so you can handle daily stress without the toxic toll it takes on your body.

There is more to life than increasing its speed.
~Mohandas K. Gandhi

CHAPTER
FOUR

Stress, the Silent Killer

Chapter Four – Stress, the Silent Killer

Take a good look around you. How many people do you see each day with frowns or stiff expressions on their faces? How many do you see with happy smiles? Not a lot of people in the second category, are there? It's understandable why the former part of the population is stressed though. People have bills to pay, kids to take care of, and a mortgage and car payment. The daily grind that characterizes the workplace only adds fuel to that ticking time bomb.

You know it and I know it. Stress is perhaps one of the most daunting and annoying maladies of our time. Whether you're a parent, a businessman or just an average Joe, you will undergo this painful condition at some point in your life. The constant pressure of life is part and parcel of living in the rat race.

Take your family for instance. They are your buffer in the most difficult situations of your life, but maintaining a balance between each family member can take a toll on anyone's patience. Top that off with your work relationships that you have to balance as well, and you have a recipe for stress.

The complex triangle is made worse when you factor in the media bombarding us with news on a daily basis. It makes the high rate of anxiety disorders we're seeing today understandable, doesn't it? In fact, anxiety disorder is the most prevalent personality disorder in the United States today.

Stress is the most pervasive malady of our time. Indeed it has been labeled as the "silent killer." Today's technology was created with a view to making our lives easier, and in many ways it does. Unfortunately, the reverse is also true. It is also making it possible for us to work around the clock and has created a new pressure to multi-task, making our lives increasingly more difficult and far more stressful. Often people don't recognize the symptoms of stress and how harmful they are until it's too late. We are plugged into our world 24/7 between cell phones and the Internet. There is very little chance for escape from the modern world and everyday stress. In fact, 90 percent of all illness and disease is stress related, according to the National Institutes of Health (NIH).

When we feel good psychologically and we have a break from stress, our brains release neuro-chemicals that make us feel good. These neuro-chemicals have a natural analgesic effect that can actually mask physical pain. However, the opposite is also true. When we're under stress, different neuro-chemistry is released, along with cortisol and epinephrine. This mix will usually go right to the weakest points of the body and create pain in those areas. Most people don't seek help until the pain shows up, not realizing that the pain was caused by hormones and neuro-chemicals emitted due to the stress response and could have been prevented.

Almost all of us have stress of some kind. Ever wonder why that job didn't get done or why you forgot to pay the rent on time? Our brains operate on that basic fight-or-flight instinct that is hardwired into us. When we get anxious or scared, our brain goes to fight-or-flight depending on the situation we find ourselves in.

This is where stress tends to get the better of us. We have stress at home, at work, over money, over time--and over many other things as well. We consider driving a car an ordinary task, but to your body there is nothing ordinary about hurtling down the highway at 70+ miles an hour with other cars and trucks cutting in alongside you.

Even ordinary tasks can cause stress in the body. Our body will react negatively by trying to flee from the stressful situation. The best case scenario is to assess the situation at hand and try to deal with it according to a decisive plan of action. However, how many people do you know who can take the time to think when they have a runaway car hurtling at them at 60 miles an hour?

You see, whenever you decide to change something in your life-

-like going on that diet you've been putting off or learning how to cook--there will always be certain triggers that displace you from that path. We are creatures of habit. Once we develop a routine, we seldom stray from it. The moment we decide to change something, stress automatically sets in. However, that stress can be worked out once you get into the habit of the new experience and embrace it. Running from problems only delays the inevitable.

The serious implications of this ailment have intrigued the medical profession for a long time. However, this community defines stress as a physical or mental stimulus that has the tendency to produce a physiological reaction, which can lead to a number of other ailments that are also physical or mental.

You see, when your body is at its healthiest, it is actually in a state of homeostasis. This means it's balanced and on a healthy and stable road. Stress can be compared to the potholes in that road, which can be triggered by fear or traumatic experiences. Having too much going on at the same time can also cause a destructive avalanche of unprocessed emotions to come tumbling down on you when you least expect it-- sometimes known as a nervous breakdown.

What many today are calling super-stress can lead to a breakdown of vast proportions. In fact, if you take stock of your life, the aches and pains and illnesses you have are most likely the direct result of some stress-induced instrument. Your brain can only take so much abuse before the body becomes unbalanced.

Stress has the annoying tendency to pick at you when you're already at your weakest and then proceeds to pick your body apart one limb at a time. Not even a single part of your body or soul is safe from this debilitating ailment. You can't just shrug it off as a bump in the road. It has to be dealt with and processed. Think about it. One stressful event can leave you feeling like you were on the receiving end of a car crash. What do you think the long-term effects of stress will be on your body?

Studies have shown that long-term stress can lead to premature aging. Once the nerves go, other physical organs can't be far behind. The heart, muscles, immune system, and joints will all fall prey once stress sinks its poisonous teeth into you.

Most people know that they are chronically stressed. What most don't know is how that chronic stress affects their life and health. Answer these important questions:

1. Where in your body do you hold or carry stress?

2. What tools have you used to try to reduce your stress?

3. Do you think that stress is an external problem or an internal response to an external problem?

4. Do you know why your brain and nervous system are called the Master Control System?

5. On a scale from 1 to 10, with 1 being minimal and 10 being maximum, where would you rate an average day of stress in your life?

If you are honest and even remotely dialed into your body, you will have to admit that you do, in fact, hold stress in a particular place in your body. For some it may be the chest area, some it is in the stomach or neck or low back or even the feet. This is important because it may have been the first time you made the connection that stress is affecting your body.

Some people have used tools to reduce their stress in the form of drugs, food and alcohol. Others may have used Pilates, yoga, chiropractic care or meditation, all in an attempt to soften or neutralize their stress. Most people think that stress is an external problem until they really think about it; and then they realize how you respond to stress is always an internal reaction--which means that, ultimately, you have control over stress and not the other way around.

When surveyed, on a scale of 1 to 10, the average person declares that a typical day of stress for them is between 7 and 8. This intense level of daily stress is what causes the neurological epidemic we are now facing. That's why it's become so important to induce a sense of normalcy into your everyday routine. This includes getting involved in stress reduction and relaxation activities on a daily basis to rediscover the normal equilibrium that a content mind and a relaxed body can give us.

Relieving stress has become a booming business. Yoga is currently a $6 billion business and ranks as one of the fastest growing industries in the country. Relaxation drinks are a $521 million business and growing fast. Massage chairs are a $250 million industry. All of these are focused on one thing--relieving your stress.

That's why we've written this book. We want to give you the tools, knowledge and skills of a mind-based and brain-based wellness program to maximize your potential and live the life you were meant to live. What if you could shed stress and be productive to your fullest capacity? Within the pages of this book you will find the solutions to strengthen your will and achieve the dreams you left at the crossroads of your destiny.

What is Brain Stress?

Since 1988 the rate of anti-depressant use in the United States has increased 400 percent. Forty million American adults are affected with an anxiety disorder. One in ten Americans aged 12 and older are taking anti-depressant medications. This is just a small slice of shocking statistics. We could probably fill half this book with more statistics just like them. What this shows is that brain stress is creating multiple forms of physical stress, which is resulting in various neurological issues and a wide range of different diseases.

It's important to realize that each and every person on earth has an inner pharmacy. We don't really need prescribed medications in many instances. We possess the most powerful pharmacy on earth--our brains. This is an incredible organ capable of releasing 30,000 different neurochemicals with a simple thought. The aim and purpose of this book is to teach you how to train your brain to think the thoughts that trigger the release of positive and healthy neurochemistry--the kind that leads to a happy and fulfilling life.

Today, for people to truly achieve wellness, we must learn to manage our stress and to cope with our ever-changing environment. We simply can't eliminate stress completely. It's too prevalent in the world around us, inherent in our tech-based, fast-paced and toxic environment. We need to teach ourselves coping mechanisms to protect us from the psychological effects of stress and to help our brains keep up with the fast-paced world we're living in--leaving our brains free to do the job the brain was designed to do.

Why Is Brain Stress So Dangerous?

More than 2 billion people worldwide currently suffer from brain-based health challenges. All forms of stress--be it stress from relationships, time, work, traffic, deadlines, health, money, or emotions--are a form of brain stress. You may not be fully aware of brain stress but everyone suffers from it at one time or another. No one is immune. We are here to offer you hope and solutions to this raging epidemic.

Periods of defense physiology, or what's known as Sympathetic Survival Syndrome, need to be followed by a recovery period in order to rebalance the brain and body chemistry. Today, people are consistently exposed to stressful situations that don't allow our bodies time for recovery. Over time, the brain begins to habituate to the stressful state and that's when we become trapped in Beta mode (a high Beta brain wave frequency)--that mode that doesn't allow for relaxation or creativity. This sets the stage for a poor quality of life, physical decline and disease to take hold.

Whenever the defense physiology kicks in, the body goes on high alert with all the reactions and responses that go with it. The heart rate, blood pressure, sugar levels and respiration rates all increase exponentially. The gastrointestinal and immune activities decrease and our pupils dilate. All of these physical reactions are useful and normal when we're faced with real stressors and the body needs to prepare for fight-or-flight to remain safe. The problem comes when we don't allow our bodies the downtime necessary to recover from this type of stress; therefore limiting our ability to recover.

Some of the latest and hottest business books on the market tell us that the most productive people are highly focused for short bursts of high performance ranging from 90 minutes to three hours. Within this window of time, there is complete focus on the problem or activity at hand. It is a high intensity, high concentration and productive time. It is then followed by a recovery period. There can be two or three "power hours" within a daily time frame, but they must be followed by an hour or two of recovery time so the brain can process and then re-engage.

This is fully consistent with what we know about exercise. The hottest trend in exercising, based on current and relevant research, is high intensity interval training. This is working at maximum capacity for short bursts of time and then having a low intensity recovery period.

Notice the importance of the recovery period for both the physical and the mental workout. The underlying problem we're seeing today is that people are not allowing for recovery time. They are not taking the time out after a high intensity situation to allow their bodies and minds to recoup. Too much fight-or-flight response without the corresponding rest and relaxation response is what distress is all about.

Both of these states, high performance and recovery, are regulated by the autonomic nervous system (ANS), and specifically, two systems within the ANS:

- The sympathetic nervous system
- The parasympathetic nervous system

The ANS regulates the functions of our internal organs such as the heart, stomach and intestines. The ANS is part of the peripheral nervous system and it also controls some of the muscles within the body.

We are usually unaware of the ANS because it functions involuntary and reflexively. For example, we do not notice when blood vessels change size or when our resting heart rate is faster than it should be. However, with the right training, many people can be taught to control some functions of the ANS such as heart rate or blood pressure.

Your sympathetic nervous system is about survival. Your parasympathetic nervous system is about healing and recovery. Your sympathetic system is involved in fight-or-flight and your parasympathetic system is about rest and digest. During the fight-or-flight response, the adrenal glands go into overdrive. This is a huge problem in today's society. This continually turned-on fight-or-flight response manifests in disease and behavioral problems rising to the epidemic proportions that we see today.

We have the ability to take the edge off and rebalance the nervous system. There are tools at our disposal that can easily and effectively allow us to bring the nervous system back into harmony, allowing recovery from Sympathetic Survival Syndrome. With the constant state of stress in our lives we need to take the time to reboot, rebalance, reset and restore harmony between the sympathetic and parasympathetic systems within our brains and nervous systems.

How is Your Nervous System Managing s\Stress?

Within the healing arts it has been well understood for years that all diseases are classified into two categories: a) a state of under activity and b) a state of over activity. Medicine's traditional approach was to develop drugs that either stimulated or depressed the system in an attempt to achieve a normal balance (homeostasis). Unfortunately, though, must drugs have side-effects that prevent homeostasis. This medical approach is still practiced today, but more and more people are now rejecting the "better health through better chemistry" that has been the focus of modern medicine for decades—and has spawned a multi-billion dollar pharmaceutical industry.

We must consider that if disease is a result of this imbalance (that is, over or under-arousal), then good health can be accomplished by creating a balanced state—and the place this happens is in the nervous system, 75 percent of which is in the brain.

The Balanced Nervous System

A balanced brain and nervous system results in good health, a state known as allostasis (adaptive balance with an appropriate return to normal) or salutogenesis (the opposite of pathogenesis which considers disease to be normal).

Allostasis and salutogenesis equal the desired states for ideal health expression. In this balanced state a person would have: present time consciousness, good recovery ability, high energy, few symptoms, resistance to infections, positive mental attitude, mental alertness, excellent health. This person looks younger than his/her years and remains active and vibrant.

We can measure the vital signs of this state by the action of the normal (actually human average) physiological responses of your body. These measurements include heart rate, respiratory rate, hand temperature, brain wave activity, heart rate variability (ratio between heart rhythm and respiratory rhythm) and skin conductance (skin moisture).

So What if it Doesn't?

This means that your system is no longer working in a state of ease. It cannot just get along with all the activities and stresses in your life without consuming more energy than normal. Energy that was destined for growth and repair now has to go to keeping everything working the best it can. Your system is now out of balance or stressed. There are four states and stages of imbalance. The states are over-aroused, under-aroused, unstable, and exhausted. The stages are mild, moderate and severe.

Stages

The stages of mild, moderate and severe apply to all of the states of dis-ease of the system. An example: take the state of over-arousal; a mild stage would show only a few of the characteristics while a severe stage would not only exhibit more characteristics but they would also be much more debilitating.

The Over-aroused State.

This state has high-energy demands. It is also the most common of the imbalanced states as a result of the stressful lifestyle of the times. When stress is prolonged, the body's responses stay in the high alert level longer than they were designed to, which creates damage to the system. The result of prolonged over-arousal includes: cold hands, tight muscles, teeth grinding, anxiety, heart palpitations, restless sleep, poor social awareness, poor comprehension, poor expression of emotion, recurrent infections, multiple competing trains of thought, high blood pressure, accelerated aging, slowed healing responses and irritable bowel. (Remember, every so-called disease is a result of either an over-stimulated or under-stimulated system).

The signs and symptoms of this over-aroused state of the body are then grouped into various combinations and given the name of a specific disease. In truth, they are nothing more than manifestations of the system being out of balance in a prolonged over-aroused state. While it is true you can treat these signs and symptoms with one form of care or another (drugs and/or surgery), the question remains – by only addressing the symptoms, are you doing anything to correct the cause?

The Under-aroused State

This state has low energy expression. If you think of depression in its classic form, then this is a picture of the body's response ability in under-arousal. It can be deceiving however, as in Attention Deficit Disorder (ADD). The misnomer of hyperactive on an ADD individual leads to a misunderstanding of the real problem. ADD individual's EEG (Electroencephalograph) does not demonstrate the over-aroused nervous system one would expect from a hyperactive response pattern. It shows just the opposite. Their nervous response is just barely awake. The only method they know, which will keep them awake and functioning, is to keep moving and active.

Ramifications of an under-aroused system are: ADD (including impulsivity, distraction and disorganization), depression, lack of motivation, poor concentration, spaciness, hypoglycemia, constipation, low pain threshold, difficulty awakening, cognitive worry, irritability, incontinence, lack of energy.

The Unstable State

Here the old simple view of the medical model of stimulate or depress treatment becomes out of date. While the concept is still valid, there is a twist in how it needs to be applied. The Unstable State includes both over and under-aroused patterns plus adds a few of its own depending on its stage. This state exhibits a higher level of imbalance than either of the above and tends to move back and forth between Over- and Under-aroused states. The system is now so stressed that any added stress creates havoc and the body's reaction can swing wildly from over to under in a short time period. This creates its own signs and symptoms beyond any of those found in the states above, which may include: migraine headaches, seizures, narcolepsy, sleepwalking, hot flashes, PMS, multiple chemical sensitivities, bed wetting, eating disorders, bi-polar disorder, mood swings and panic attacks. People with wide ranges of health challenges would fall into this state of imbalance.

The Exhausted State

This is the most dangerous of all. It is automatically in the severe stage. The system is now into chaos existence mode. It is so over-stressed that body systems are no longer able to work in harmony. This can be so severe the body systems start attacking each other. Its own communication system is in such disarray that messages and responses no longer match. Unchecked it will be life ending. Health challenges include: all of those listed in Over-aroused plus conditions such as Chronic Fatigue Syndrome, Epstein–Barr Syndrome, M.S., Fibromyalgia, Cancer.

In a later chapter we'll be discussing the benefits of chiropractic for brain health, but it's the same chiropractic you've heard about or previously experienced. We're talking about Neurologically Based Chiropractic (NBC) wherein the chiropractor works with your nervous system to restore your health.

Today, there is technology that can measure the state of your nervous system in normal mode, in stress mode and in recovery mode. It can show you why you are experiencing your health challenges and it can help the doctor design a program of care to help restore your normal allostatic balance.

If you are in the unstable group, it is very important that you tell your chiropractor your neurological state at each visit before care begins. (Examples: "Bright-eyed and bushy-tailed," or "Sleep monster just won't let go.")

This is not about treating a disease, as that is not what chiropractors do. Medicine treats disease. Chiropractic's intent is to help your nervous system return to a healthy balanced state, a state of ease, by removing interference and retraining normal patterns of reaction.

The job of an NBC doctor is to access your nervous system and either stimulate it or depress it by means of a chiropractic adjustment, restoring it to the wonderful normal state of balance. NBC doctors are also able to offer additional re-training methods to augment the power of the chiropractic adjustment in this restoration.

To really see how your system is working, an NBC doctor will want to place your system under stress; watch how your system handles it; then see if it is able to recover and reset your normal levels quickly. All of this can be determined with the NeuroInfiniti biofeedback system in about 15 minutes.

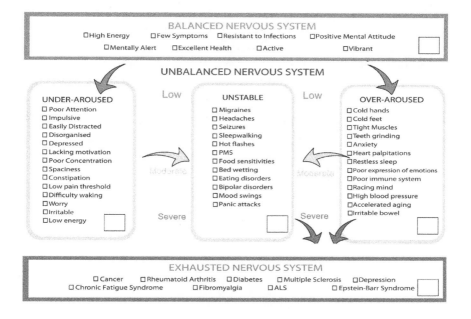

This BIOCHART will help you determine where you think you are based on how you feel and the health challenges you are facing. You may be mostly in one area but find yourself in several of these states. If you find yourself in the latter group then you will most likely be in the unstable group. If however, you are in the exhausted state, you need to talk about your choices and additional methods to help you get stabilized. This is a serious state and needs care and understanding.

If you are concerned about the state of your nervous system and would like to have an assessment done, please call the offices of Dr. Richard Barwell DC, creator of the NeuroInfiniti stress measurement tool, at 877-233-0022 and ask for a referral to a Neurologically Based Chiropractic doctor near you.

A Simple but Profound Summary

All forms of stress are brain stress. When the brain is stressed, it goes out of balance and, unfortunately, the body follows and goes out of balance as well. This shows up as illness, disease, behavioral problems, loss of vitality and rapid aging. When the brain is balanced again, fortunately, the body will follow. We call this healing.

"When you arise in the morning, think of what a precious privilege it is to be alive--to breathe, to think, to enjoy, to love."

--Marcus Aurelius

CHAPTER
FIVE
The Heart-Brain Connection

CHAPTER FIVE : The Heart-Brain Connection

The last two decades have witnessed the recognition of a significant relationship between the autonomic nervous system and cardiovascular activity. Heart Rate Variability (HRV) is a measure of the naturally-occurring beat-to-beat changes in heart rate/heart rhythms. It serves as a critical method for gauging human health and resiliency.

Numerous studies show HRV is a key indicator of physiological resiliency and behavioral flexibility, and can reflect an ability to adapt effectively to stress and environmental demands.

The ability to effectively adapt is central to health and wellbeing and a foundational pillar of chiropractic philosophy. When we have the ability to adapt to our internal and external stressors in a timely fashion, we are in a state of ease. When we lose the ability to effectively adapt, we move into a state of dis-ease, and when we remain in a state of dis-ease long enough, we eventually become diseased.

"The study of heart rate variability," according to HeartMath's signature work, Science of the Heart, "is a powerful, objective and noninvasive tool to explore the dynamic interactions between physiological, mental, emotional and behavioral processes."

Researchers use HRV, as measured by an electrocardiogram (ECG) or pulse wave recording, to assess the state of the autonomic nervous system (ANS), which controls our heart and breath rates, gastrointestinal tract movement and gland secretion among other internal bodily functions. Several innovators in the field have utilized HRV analysis for many years to examine the influence positive and negative emotions have on the ANS.

Many people are surprised to learn that the heart actually sends more information to the brain than the brain sends to the heart via the ANS, and that the rhythmic patterns produced by the heart directly affect the brain's ability to process information, including decision-making, problem-solving and creativity. They also directly affect how we feel and function.

It is well known that mental and emotional states directly affect the activity of the ANS. A number of studies have shown that HRV is an important indicator of both physiological resiliency and behavioral flexibility, reflecting an individual's capacity to adapt effectively to stress and environmental demands. In short, HRV is a measure of autonomic function.

In order to achieve brain-based wellness, it is important and necessary to achieve and maintain a harmonious and balanced relationship between the heart and the brain. This type of relationship is referred to as coherence, which occurs when a constructive waveform produced by two or more waves are in phase or frequency locked. In physiology, the term is used to describe a state in which two or more of the body's oscillatory systems, such as respiration and heart rhythm patterns become synchronous and operate at the same frequency. This type of coherence is called entrainment.

Here are some key points to consider as researched and documented by the Institute of HeartMath:

• The cells of the amygdala (an almond shaped set of cells located deep in the brain that is associated with emotions, emotional behavior and motivation) synchronize with the heart with each heartbeat.
• We can better regulate our emotions by learning how to self-regulate our heart rhythms.
• Getting our heart and brain working together will optimize our mental, physical and emotional health.
• The heart helps to power and direct the brain.
• The rhythmic patterns of the beating heart neurologically affect our brain function and when it does, we call that integration.
• Studies suggest that focusing on positive emotions of love, gratitude and joy leads to important integrative states of brain function.

- Positive emotions are a tonic for heart-brain health and wellbeing.
- By self-regulating your positive emotions along with your breathing, you can positively influence your heart and brain.
- The heart sends more information to the brain then the brain sends to your heart as 90-95 percent of the nerves connecting the heart and brain are afferent, meaning they convey impulses toward the central nervous system.
- The heart's electrical charge is 60 times greater in amplitude than the brain's and the magnetic field of the heart is 100 times stronger than the magnetic field produced by the brain.
- The heart is the most powerful generator of rhythm information patterns in the body.
- Heart coherence is the state where the heart-brain interactions, mind, emotions and nervous system are operating in sync and in energetic cooperation.
- When we are stressed, the hearts rhythms become erratic and disorderly creating an incoherent waveform.
- Heart rate variability (HRV) is the physiological phenomenon of variation in the time between heartbeats. It is measured in the beat-to-beat interval.

In a later chapter, utilizing the HeartQuest, widely considered the most advanced HRV technology to date, we'll be looking at inspiring before and after HRV images that support the benefits that can be achieved with the Brain-Based Wellness modalities outlined in this book, often in twenty minutes or less.

CHAPTER

SIX

THE BRAIN WAVES
Beta, Alpha, Theta and Delta

Chapter Six:
THE BRAIN WAVES-- Beta, Alpha, Theta and Delta

We've mentioned your brain wave patterns several times throughout the preceding pages. So let's discuss what those brain waves are and why they matter.

It's been confirmed by a number of scientists that the brain is, indeed, an electrochemical organ. It has been discovered that it can actually generate ten watts of electrical power on its own. This occurs in specific parts of the human brain and occurs in the form of brain waves, which are divided into four categories according to their frequency levels.

What are Brainwaves?

Your brain is made up of billions of brain cells called neurons, which use electricity to communicate with each other. The combination of millions of neurons sending signals at once produces an enormous amount of electrical activity in the brain, which can be detected using sensitive medical equipment (such as an EEG), measuring electricity levels over areas of the scalp.

The combination of electrical activity of the brain is commonly called a brain wave pattern, because of its cyclic, "wave-like" nature.

Brainwave Frequencies

With the discovery of brain waves came the discovery that electrical activity in the brain will change depending on what the person is doing. For instance, the brain waves of a sleeping person are vastly different than the brain waves of someone wide-awake. Over the years, more sensitive equipment has brought us closer to figuring out exactly what brainwaves represent and with that, what they mean about a person's health and state of mind.

There are four primary brain wave frequencies: Beta, Alpha, Theta and Delta. Today, most people spend nearly all their waking time in just one—Beta, the only brain wave where stress, pain, fear and frustration exist.

Beta Waves

Beta is the frequency in play when we are reactionary. It's called the reactionary mind. Beta is the normal state of alertness. We need it to be able to drive a car or read an instruction manual. In fact, we need it to do anything that requires conscious attention.

Don't you feel more energized when you're actively participating or involved in mental activities like speeches and debates? That's because your brain's Beta waves are working full throttle to help you. These brain waves are of relatively low amplitude but are the fastest of all the brainwaves. Beta brain waves are typical of a strong and fully awake and engaged mind.

However, this is also the brain wave frequency that allows for fear, anger, frustration or negative thinking. In fact, we can only experience pain in Beta mode and it is the only brain wave where negative emotions are even possible. That makes this the brain state that is hardest to make changes in. When the brain gets out of balance and we have high levels of Beta waves, it represses the normal function of the other waves in our brain that allow us to wind down, relax, be joyful or creative.

A lot of people today have trouble falling asleep because they go to bed in Beta mode, when we need to be switching to Alpha mode at this time.

Alpha Waves

Alpha waves come after Beta waves in order of frequency and are the opposite of the latter. They are usually slower but higher in amplitude, since their frequency ranges from 9-14 cycles per second. This brainwave is generated when, for instance, you sit down to rest after completing a chore. Meditation can also generate these brain waves.

When we first start to fall asleep, we switch into predominantly Alpha mode. We call this the intuitive mind. Once we're in Alpha mode we're in a state of relaxation or light meditation. Alpha mode is associated with quiet times in our lives when we're involved in creative pursuits, meditation or prayer.

If you have a favorite hobby or craft that you often get lost in, you're likely generating primarily Alpha waves at that time. The same is true if you're having a pleasant daydream, fantasizing about an upcoming vacation, or simply in a quiet, contemplative mood.

If your brain is functioning properly, the Alpha waves flow into Theta waves as you fall sleep.

Theta Waves

These brainwaves are capable of greater amplitude but demonstrate lower frequency as compared to the previous two, with a range of 5-8 cycles per second. You usually experience them while daydreaming after completing a task. The best example would be of someone driving to work on a regular basis. It's not surprising for such a person to forget the last few miles they drove once they reach their destination. This is when Theta waves are working on their mind.

Theta mode is the intuitive part of your mind. It's the activity of the brain that can help you solve the problems in your life. You may have heard stories of great inventors who intentionally go to sleep with a problem posed on their minds and they awake with the solution in hand. They got a brief peek into what we refer to as the super-conscious part of their minds.

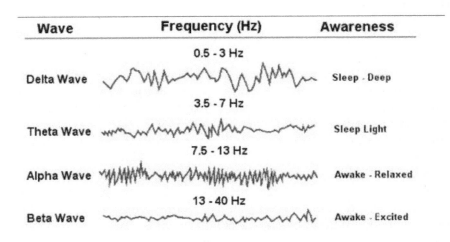

Wave	Frequency (Hz)	Awareness
Delta Wave	0.5 - 3 Hz	Sleep - Deep
Theta Wave	3.5 - 7 Hz	Sleep Light
Alpha Wave	7.5 - 13 Hz	Awake - Relaxed
Beta Wave	13 - 40 Hz	Awake - Excited

Proper brain wave activity is essential to good health, both mentally and physically. The brain needs to go through these brain wave states every day and it especially needs time to allow the Alpha and Theta states to work properly. The problem is most people spend little to no time in the Alpha and Theta modes. They have trained themselves to deal with stress with the reactionary mind alone, in Beta mode. In other words, they're reacting to life instead of living it.

Moreover, when we don't sleep properly, our brains don't spend enough time in the Alpha and Theta modes, and therefore, cannot recharge properly. Those who snore may be interested to know that snoring prevents the brain from going through the proper sleep cycles. Instead of going from Beta to Alpha and then to Theta to get to Delta (which is deep sleep), it tries to skip from Beta to Delta, skipping the Alpha and Theta stages.

Think of Alpha and Theta as the time for doing paperwork in the brain. It's when the brain stores, categorizes and organizes the day's activities so things that are meaningful and useful are systematically encoded and organized in a way that your subconscious can access them for future use. Trying to do everything in Beta mode is almost like saying, "I want to have a great business but I'm not going to do any of the paperwork that comes with it." Common sense tells us that that won't work. We simply can't learn or remember in Beta mode. We need the Alpha and Theta modes to properly process the information that we've gathered throughout our day. This is why people under extreme stress have poor memories and muddled thinking. They're stuck in Beta mode and aren't processing that information.

Delta Waves

The last brain wave, Delta waves, have the greatest amplitude but also the lowest frequency out of all the brainwaves. Typically they range from 1.4-4 cycles per second. These brain waves never reach zero--you would be considered brain dead if they did. You can usually experience Delta waves up to 2-3 cycles per second during a dreamless sleep.

Delta is the deep sleep state, a state we all need to reach so that the body can rebuild, repair, renew and otherwise access the innate intelligence that keeps our bodies functioning.

Sometimes, however, people are generating a lot of Delta activity while awake. This is a sure sign of exhaustion. The brain is attempting to sleep while you're trying to think, learn, remember or participate in activities. Needless to say, this dichotomy doesn't work for anyone, and it's the reason people who don't get enough sleep also suffer from brain fog and memory loss.

Did you know that before the invention of electricity people slept an average of ten hours a night? However, today people are getting far less. In a survey conducted by the hotel company Travelodge, 65 percent are sleeping an average of just six hours and 27 minutes every night.

That's over 30 minutes less than today's general recommendation that adults get seven to nine hours of slumber a night. Get less on a regular basis and you put yourself at risk for a whole host of health consequences that range from bothersome to fatal, including memory and heart problems, increased cancer and diabetes risk and earlier death.

As you can see, all four brain wave modes are extremely important for proper functioning. Beta mode is our wide-awake, reactionary state that we live in most often. Delta is the other end of the spectrum where deep sleep allows us to repair and rest for the upcoming day. We also need those times between awake and asleep, the Alpha and Theta modes. Whether it's through mindful meditation, relaxation, yoga, painting or fishing by a stream, massage or chiropractic, to live a happy, balanced life you need those periods when your brain gets a chance to tap into these essential mid-point brain waves.

Meditation is a really important technique to help us get out of Beta and into Alpha and Theta modes. Many people find it extremely helpful in calming their minds and dealing with the stresses of life. Later on we're going to introduce you to an alternative to meditation; a way to rapidly and dramatically get the results of meditation in a much more powerful state and much more quickly. There is truly some amazing technology out there that can help us overcome the effects of our overloaded lifestyles.

The Conscious and Unconscious Mind

Besides the four brain wave patterns, you also have two states of mind--the conscious and the unconscious, which are responsible for everything you think about and feel. The former accounts for approximately 8 percent of your mind's thinking process and is what is actually aware of your surroundings at any given moment in time. It is also responsible for storing your memories, as well as making logic-based decisions such as balancing your checkbook or writing an email. In other words, the conscious mind makes us aware of who we are.

You may be surprised to find out that the other 92 percent belongs to that part of your mind that comprises the real you. This other-than-conscious part of your mind is responsible for storing data from almost every experience or thought you've had, which is then made manifest in the form of your beliefs and values, as well as your self-image. You perceive the world through this potent amalgamation of thoughts and feelings--thus creating your world view out of it.

This part of your brain works on its own without asking for conscious effort on your part. Wondering where you got that mind-boggling idea from? The unconscious mind is the part of your mind that houses your imagination, emotions and creativity, which is why you can recall a past memory and relish it as if it were happening in the present, or imagine yourself as a bird in flight without ever leaving the ground.

There are a limitless number of incredible things you can do when your brain is in balance and you have the right mindset to do it with. In the pages that follow, you'll learn simple strategies for rekindling the same balance of brain wave activity—what we call full-spectrum brainwave activity—that we all had as kids, when we were free from stress, had unbridled creativity and photographic memories.

Using the HRV equipment dicussed earlier, we will show you the results for Jennifer a 39 year old mother of an Autistic child. We typically see 20-30% neurological improvement with the MindFit or chiropractic care. What you will see in the following pages is nothing short of astonishing. You will see how Jennifer's nervous system is able to adjust to the therapies. Jennifer's "Stress Index" went from a 475 to a 303 with her SMT MindFit Session. Her "Vital Force" went from 28 to 44. This figure represents her energy level.

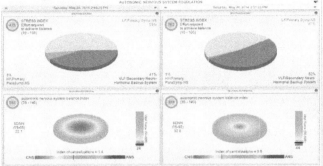

Jenifer's "Stress Index" went from a 303 to a 147 after her chiropractic adjustment.

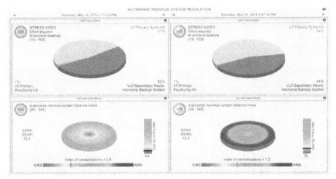

Her "Vital Force" went from 44 to 75. These numers are significant as you can see in the panel below this represents an over 200% improvement by lowering stress and increasing her vital energy.

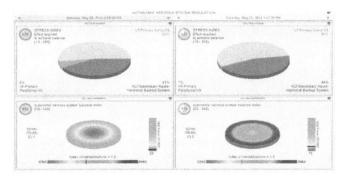

Here we see Jennifer's nervous system and how it is regulating. We can see she went from 9% to 29% in Autonomic, 31% to 61% in Neuro-Hormonal, Cardio-Vascular went from 20% to 39% and her Psycho-Emotional went from 32% to 60%

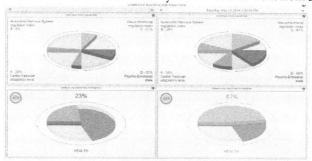

during her SMT MindFit session. Below we see how the chiropractic adjust was able to boost her numbers to 47% in Autonomic, 68% in Neuro-Hormonal, 60% in Cardio-Vascular and her Psycho-Emotional went to 60%.

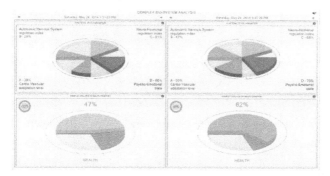

You can see in the panel below how her overall function went from 23% to 62% in about a half-hours time.

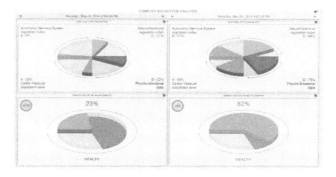

In the next three panels you will see how the brain-based approach has improved her heart's coherences. This represents how the brain is communicating with the body. You can see Jennifer started with a Coherence of 20 before her SMT MindFit session and was able to bring it up to a 39. You can also see she started the session at a biological age of 50 years and was able to bring that down to 43 year old.

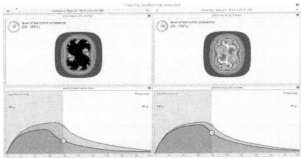

In this next panel you will see how chiropractic was able to bring her into the normal zone at 60 and bring her biological age of 39. It's important to note here

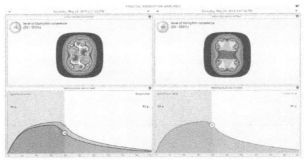

that this is all being done within the same therapeutic session. Below you will see the panel where we combine the two therapies.

On this page we show the panels describing brain wave activity and Jenifer's

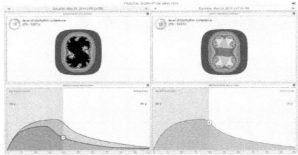

Psycho-emotional index. With her first SMT MindFit session she went from a 32 (normal is between 50-100) to a 50. It's not uncommon to see patients coming in with more Delta brain waves. This is usually a sign of poor sleeping habits. We need to remember this is the mother of an autistic child, so she is fatigued and not sleeping well. The MindFit session is working to awaken her brain and get her to activate more Alpha and Beta which in balance gives us energy to accomplish our daily goals.

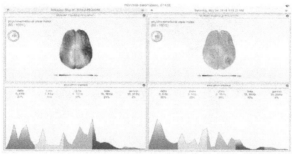

Below you will see how the chiropractic adjustment completed this for Jennifer. The adjustment boosted her psycho-emotional index all the way to 73 and her

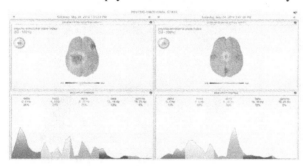

Delta is decreased to 13%. While we still don't see the amount of Beta we would like to see, Jennifer is on her way with continued treatment. Below you can see the combined benefits of the brain-based approach to wellness.

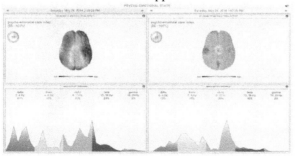

These next panels will demonstrate how the nervous system being out of balance has caused such a problem in the area of weight gain arround the world. You can see how the SMT MindFit session inproved neuro-hormonal regulation going from a 31 to 61. You can also notice her metabolic energy went from 83 to 146 and switched her from fat storage mode to fat buring mode. And this all happened while she relaxed and trained her brain.

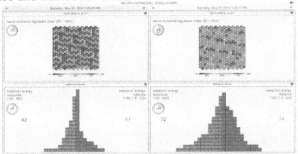

You can see in the panel below how her chiropractic adjustment really supercharges her metabolisim. boosting it to 68 on the neuro-hormonal regulation

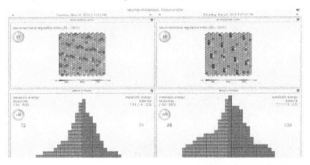

and 207 metabolic energy resources. And look at how the combination really sets Jenifer up to use the energy she has available and transform her body into a fat burning machine. Below you can see the total of the combined therapy.

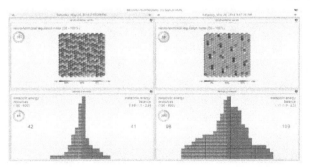

CHAPTER
SEVEN

Adjusting Your Thinking and Adjusting Your Life

Chapter Seven
Adjusting Your Thinking and Adjusting Your Life

Most people know that chiropractic care works extremely well at correcting and improving structural problems, but did you know that its real value comes from normalizing and maximizing brain function? As we have discussed previously, when the brain balances so does the body—and that is called healing.

Most people don't understand the difference between medical care and chiropractic care or realize that there is a fundamental need for both.

If you are injured or in an accident, you'll visit an emergency room where a specially-trained physician repairs the injury. He or she will set the bone, close the wound, stop the bleeding, and do whatever else is needed to save your life. If you get bit by a rattlesnake, get rabies or are exposed to bacterial meningitis, there are drugs that can save your life. Both of these scenarios are emergency situations where your body's defenses have been attacked and overwhelmed and you would die without intervention. Medical care helps your body get stabilized until it can fend for itself again.

However, in the case of chronic diseases like arthritis, diabetes, asthma, chronic disease, fibromyalgia, cancer, heart disease—actually just about 99.9% of all the diseases we know of today, the problem is essentially the same, a chronic issue developed gradually from inside out because of a functional imbalance. Your cells were unable to maintain balance because the coordinating signals were off.

Many mistakenly think of doctors of chiropractic as "back doctors" when in truth, chiropractors use the vertebra of the spine as their gateway to effect neurological balance, harmony and vibrancy. In other words, chiropractic adjustments harmonize the coordinating signals in the body.

Chiropractic care has withstood the test of time. Founded in 1895, the profession continues to make remarkable progress in its science, art and philosophy as well as its application to help patients live a better life.

More than 100 years ago in the first book written about chiropractic, D.D. Palmer, the founder of chiropractic, stated that, "life is the expression of tone." In that simple sentence is the basic principle of chiropractic. Tone is the normal degree of nerve tension. Tone is expressed in functions by normal elasticity, activity, strength and excitability of the various organs, as observed in a state of health. Consequently, the cause of disease is any variation of tone - nerves too tense or too slack.

Vertebral subluxation is the central defining clinical principle of the chiropractic profession because subluxation of the vertebrae of the spine is what alters, disturbs and distorts the normal tone of the nervous system.

As a result of new technology, clinical research and professional advancements, we now realize that the correction of the vertebral subluxation through a specific chiropractic adjustment actually normalizes and maximizes brain function.

In fact, the corrective chiropractic adjustment normalizes the tone of the entire nervous system allowing the body to heal from above-down and from inside-out. By stimulating and balancing the nervous system, doctors of chiropractic can improve the function of both the brain and the body. At the end of this chapter, you'll see images from the HeartQuest HRV and the NeuroInfiniti that demonstrate the dramatic effect a single chiropractic adjustment can make on the body's vital systems.

Chiropractors have known for years that the chiropractic adjustment is important for overall health, vitality and wellbeing.

There are increasing amounts of research to back up these claims. The field of chiropractic was founded on the idea that when vertebrae are misaligned or subluxated they put pressure on the nerves, which decreases the nerve's ability to transmit signals to the brain and the rest of the body.

Sadly, many people don't realize the powerful and positive benefits of chiropractic care. They only focus on the pain relief aspect of chiropractic. Research shows the benefits of chiropractic adjustments only begin with pain relief.

We have discovered that the brain can change for better or for worse as it adapts. This is called neuroplasticity. Neuroplasticity is the brain's ability to reorganize itself by forming new neurological connections. Negative neuroplasticity causes us to deteriorate, get sick and grow old prematurely. Positive neuroplasticity leads to improved cognitive functions, improved memory, elevated mood and optimized healing.

The overall purpose of regular chiropractic adjustments is and always has been to remove stress on the nervous system, which causes negative neuroplasticity, and to encourage positive neuroplasticity so that the body can adapt in ways to improve healing and restore normal function. Chiropractic adjustments reboot, defrag, synchronize and harmonize brain function. Chiropractic adjustments erase and neutralize chronic stress before it causes long-term damage to the brain and body

The intent of chiropractic is not necessarily to move vertebrae that are out of place back into alignment. That is a wonderful side effect, but the real intent behind any chiropractic adjustment is to restore proper communication between brain and body by improving nerve function so the body can heal itself. The main purpose is to normalize and maximize brain function.

Corrective chiropractic adjustments interrupt the current inappropriate neurological pattern that is causing deterioration, disease and disharmony. Getting adjusted with some frequency over time also will reestablish a new normal and far more appropriate neurological pattern, creating healing, health, energy, vibrancy and wellbeing.

A proper chiropractic adjustment creates a functional reorganization in the brain and makes the connections between brain cells more robust. In addition, the adjustments will improve cortical function and balance, risk evaluation, language skills, motivation, thinking, memory and overall quality of life while reducing your stress level, inflammation, muscle tone and pain. If any new drug could claim a fraction of these benefits, it would quickly become the best selling drug of all time, but we know that no such drug exists. Even more impressive, proper chiropractic care correctly administered is free from negative side effects.

This is the reason why the chiropractic profession continues to flourish and thrive with either no publicity or bad publicity, no government funding for its research, independent colleges and universities, and no drug company or insurance company spending millions or billions driving patients into our offices.

The profession grows because of one simple and profound reason: It works to improve the quality and quantity of life for millions of patients. It is our experience that people fall into one of two categories relating to chiropractic care. They either swear by us or swear at us. The number swearing by us is growing each and every day and the group swearing at us, when questioned, rarely have any understanding as to what doctors of chiropractic do, why they do what they do, or even their training and background.

It is clearly time to fully realize that better health through better chemistry is a belief system that has failed. Now is the time to transition to a new and improved belief system based on better health through better living.

Dr. Thomas Insel of The National Institute for Mental Health has said, "The unfortunate reality is that current medications help too few people to get better and very few to get well." He also has been quoted as saying, "We need to stop thinking about mental disorders and start understanding them as brain disorders."

Nobel Prize recipient Dr. Roger Sperry says, "The spine is the motor that drives the brain," and that, "Ninety percent of the stimulation and nutrition to the brain is generated by the movement of the spine." Sperry's award-winning research makes the rock solid connection between chiropractic adjustments, vertebral subluxation and brain function. When a vertebra is subluxated—the International Chiropractors Association states that the vertebral subluxation is the result of spinal bones with improper motion or position affecting nerve communication between your brain and body. They also state that the subluxation is a stress response—it loses its normal motion and weakens the spines ability to drive brain function.

Sperry's research went on to state, "Only 10 percent of our brain's energy goes into thinking, metabolism, immunity and healing because 90 percent goes into processing and maintaining the body's relationship with gravity."

Maintaining the body's relationship to gravity is known as posture. By and large, society ignores the importance of posture, to its detriment. Posture is a reflection of the stress on your brain and nervous system. Posture is a neurological program. We've all been told more times than we would like to admit to stand up straight or sit up straight; and we do momentarily, but always revert back to our poor posture as soon as we stop consciously overriding the neurological program. Posture and a misaligned/subluxated spine is a clear reflection of brain function and the best gateway to changing and improving brain function and overall health and wellbeing.

When we develop or maintain poor posture, it is a signal that your brain and nervous system are under stress. The spine is the best reflection of brain function and the best gateway to changing and improving brain function. Why is this so important? The brain coordinates everything that happens in the body.

Dr. Candace Pert, author of *Molecules of Emotion*, and a well-respected Molecular Biologist said, "How we experience our world is governed in large part by the structure and function of our brains and nervous systems."

The brain is responsible for sending messages to every organ and tissue in the body through the nervous system. Regular chiropractic care improves the brain's ability to transmit its messages and stay healthy, because when the brain is balanced, the body will always follow. This is called healing.

Chiropractic is one of the only wellness practices that focus on improving not only physical function but mental function and brain health as well. The adjustment is specifically designed to remove interference to normal functioning—reducing, and with regular care, eliminating the negative effects of stress on the brain. Brain balance and homeostasis can be re-established in the body in several ways: deep meditation, rhythmic breathing, exercise, being in nature, laughter, deep Delta sleep; and of course, regular chiropractic care.

Manual manipulation of the spine and other joints in the body has been around for centuries. Hippocrates, the famous Greek physician who lived from 460-357 BC, published a text detailing the importance of manual manipulation. In one of his writings he declares, "Get knowledge of the spine, for this is the requisite for many diseases." Evidence of manual manipulation of the body has been found among the ancient civilizations of Egypt, Babylon, Syria, Japan, the Incas, Mayans and native Americans."

The understanding of the human frame or structure and its

relationship to human function or health has been around since ancient times and is best described by the famous Thomas Edison quote, "The doctor of the future will give no medicine, but will interest his patients in the care of the human frame, in diet, and in the cause and prevention of disease." (From *Discover Wellness...How Staying Healthy Can Make You Rich*, By Dr. Jason Deitch and Dr. Bob Hoffman)

Chiropractic is the best-kept secret in health care, but now you know why a doctor of chiropractic should be on your wellness team. In fact, many chiropractors see themselves as the CWO, which stands for Chief Wellness Officer, who can professionally guide you to make better educated decisions on how to get well and stay well without the side effects of drugs.

Recent scientific research is demonstrating what practitioners have known for many years—that chiropractic benefits the whole body and brain, not just the back as many people believe. We will examine some of these research studies below.

As we have discussed previously, neuroplasticity is the brain's ability to form new neural pathways in relation to new circumstances. People are familiar with negative neuroplasticity in the form of memory loss or mental decline. One of the most effective ways to improve neuroplasticity is through regular and corrective chiropractic adjustment.

The brain and nervous system control all the functions in our bodies—literally every function of every organ and cell of your body including breathing, balance, blood pressure, digestion and more. When your brain functions well, your entire body functions well. The more stress we place our bodies under, the faster decline happens. If nothing is done to alleviate this stress, it will be continually reinforced.

Chiropractic care focuses on removing stress on the nervous system, which would otherwise contribute to mental and physical decline. The chiropractic adjustment is designed specifically to remove interference to normal health. With regular chiropractic care, the stresses of daily life that can cause mental decline can be reversed. Proper chiropractic care creates a functional reorganization in the brain and makes the connections between cells more robust. It interrupts inappropriate neurological patterns, reduces our stress levels, as well as reducing inflammation and pain.

To demonstrate this, let's take a look at a study done by Arlene Welch and Ralph Boone published in the Journal of Chiropractic Medicine, September 2008, regarding the positive effects of cervical chiropractic adjustments. In this study, the authors theorized that if an adjustment were performed on certain parts of the spine, certain responses in the body would occur. The study examined 40 volunteers who had no history of heart disease. Each of the 40 participants was evaluated over five visits over a two-week period and each was evaluated pre- and post-observation.

During the study, the results showed that while pulse rate did not vary significantly pre- and post-adjustment, diastolic blood pressure dropped significantly among participants receiving cervical (neck) adjustments. Diastolic pressure is associated with hypertension, so being able to lower this number can be beneficial to patients because pulse pressure is a risk factor for heart disease and premature death.

This particular study demonstrates that depending on where a chiropractor adjusts a patient there are shifts in the way the body alters the sympathetic (the body's internal systems, survival) and parasympathetic (homeostasis and balance, healing) responses.

We know that imbalance between our sympathetic and parasympathetic nervous systems is the cause of nearly all disease— physically and mentally. When the brain goes out of balance, the body will follow and go out of balance. We call this sickness and disease. It is important to understand that our sympathetic nervous system is primarily about survival while our parasympathetic nervous system is primarily about healing. When we are in survival mode, our ability to heal, grow and learn is greatly reduced. When the brain is out of balance, we can't live healthy or optimally. Ongoing chiropractic adjustment makes great strides in balancing the body and the brain— reducing risk of disease and physical ailment.

Another study presented at The Sherman College of Straight Chiropractic found that chiropractic adjustment has a positive effect on the central nervous system, including the four brain waves. This important study was a result of research conducted by Dr. Richard Barwell, a well-known and highly-respected chiropractor, along with psychologists and biofeedback experts, Annette Long, Ph.D. and Alvah Byers, Ph.D.

As discussed earlier, brain wave function is measured on the four frequencies of Alpha, Beta, Theta and Delta. Alpha waves reflect meditative and healing states, Beta is your active and awake brain. Theta is light sleep and relaxation; and Delta is deep sleep where the body repairs itself and energy is replenished.

This study was conducted over a three-year period using 100 study participants. They were examined with EEG before and after chiropractic adjustment. The EEG scans showed improvement in all areas of brain function post adjustment. Particularly, the researchers noticed increases in the Alpha brain wave patterns post adjustment. These brain wave patterns are associated with relaxation, health and healing. Also, interesting to note, some of the 100 participants who already had balanced brain function pre-adjustment showed no negative effects resulting from chiropractic adjustment.

So what is the end conclusion? It was demonstrated that the brain and nervous system are essential to all functions in the body. A stressed brain leads to dysfunction in the body. Chiropractic care is essential to removing the stress and restoring healthy function not only physically but also mentally.

In perhaps one of the most groundbreaking studies done to date, award-winning researcher Dr. Heidi Haavik-Taylor demonstrated that chiropractic care sends signals to the brain that changes the way the brain controls muscles in the body.

Dr. Haavik-Taylor says, "The process of a spinal adjustment is like rebooting a computer. The signals that these adjustments send to the brain, via the nervous system, resets muscle behavior patterns."

Dr. Haavik-Taylor spent years researching the effects of chiropractic adjustment on the nervous system—actually measuring brain waves before and after adjustment. It was shown that when participants were measured pre- and post-adjustment, there was a positive shift in brain wave activity to a more balanced and relaxed brain wave state.

Based on her findings, Dr. Haavik-Taylor believes that stimulating the nervous system via chiropractic adjustment improves the function of the entire body—something chiropractors have known for years. Now, there is scientific proof to back up their claims.

Similarly, in a study conducted by Brian Mahaffrey, DC, on a 26-year old male patient who exhibited no pain or symptoms prior to adjustment, it was found that chiropractic adjustment decreased the imbalances in thermal readings of skin temperature done pre- and post-adjustment. Dr. Mahaffrey's conclusion based on his study was that reducing subluxations in the spine immediately has a positive impact on neurological function.

Here is a quote we love because it really sums this up: "Align the brain and the body. Your brain is the control system of the body. Brain balance and harmony is essential to overall wellbeing and optimal cognitive, emotional and physical performance. Once the brain is balanced, the body always follows. This condition of harmony is known as homeostasis. Once you achieve homeostasis, you will enjoy new states of self-regulation and relaxation, allowing you to think more clearly, perform more successfully and experience a higher degree of hope and happiness."

As you can see from just a few of the numerous studies—and there are many more that can be found with a simple Google search—the benefits of chiropractic go far beyond mere pain relief or accident rehabilitation. Regular use of chiropractic care is important in reducing brain stress, in maintaining your nervous system function and thereby maintaining brain health and reducing the incidences of memory loss and encouraging positive neuroplasticity and peak healing in the brain. If you are not currently utilizing chiropractic care as part of your wellness lifestyle, it is time to start!

Next we'll be discussing, brainwave entrainment technology, the high-tech solution. We consider chiropractic care the high-touch solution. High-tech and high-touch perfectly complement one another. We have been researching and studying the healing effects of chiropractic care and brainwave entrainment together and the results have been truly amazing. Better, faster and longer lasting results than either one alone.

You can certainly improve your health, reduce your stress and rebalance your brain using either; but the one-two punch of using both on an ongoing basis may very well be the smartest decision you can ever make for lowering your stress, balancing and enhancing your brain and living the life you were meant to live with energy, joy and fulfillment.

• Stress in life is really about your ability to adapt to your environment. The better you are able to adapt the less stress your systems face. The role of the nervous system in this ability to adapt is the critical factor regarding your health status. Current research states that 95% of all illness directly involves stress factors.

• Other recent research has shown an important point that was not clearly understood in the past. This was that while chiropractic care has a great history of good responses in a wide range of health challenges, the historical position of a misaligned vertebra pressing on a spinal nerve and the correction of the misalignment was the reason for the results wasn't the real facts. Today we have better information and research to be able to understand why the Chiropractic adjustment works so well in improving so many health issues. Today we know that Chiropractic adjustment help the brain reset itself to a better balance which in turn brings the body's system in to better balance.

• The Stress Response Evaluation (SRE) seen here shows exactly this. First, note the charts with the red and green bars. This is called the "patient report". You see the "S" and "R" under each of the headers – the "S" stands for what the heart (for example) was doing during the stressor part of the test, the "R" stand for what the heart was doing during recovery. Above 0 or green is ideal. The higher the number the more the stress on the system. Now compare the post care chart. Note the vast improvement across the entire group of systems.

• The other chart show us in detail exactly how different parts of the brain handle different types of stressors and how they recover once the stressor is gone. The top set of bars reveal what is happening in the cortex region while the bottom 6 boxes show how the limbic system is working.

• The best way to understand these is to simply look at the ideal chart and compare each box in this scan. While there is great improvement and the person is feeling much better, it is easy to see that more correction is needed to bring the system to an ideal function level. Health is when all the system work within their ideal ranges of stress responses and then recover.

• The role of the cortex - The cortex of the brain is the outside portion of the brain made up of cells called neurons. The neurons form a wiring network that controls and coordinates all the rest of your body's functions. Your memories are stored in these networks with an emotional tag. Ninety-eight percent (98%) of your brain activity is at the subconscious level, so an external event can trigger a response in your brain that you will not be aware of consciously. The Stress Response Evaluation (SRE) shows how you respond and/or recover from different stressors. Our goal is to determine the state of your cortical activity and work out a plan to reset and retrain it to ideal function.

• The cortex patterns - Your brain operates best in a balanced state. This means you would have the ability to create Beta focus when called for under stress and dial it out when no longer needed. At the same time you need to be able to create the relaxation recovery brain activity in order for healing and growth. These include Alpha, Theta and Delta brain wave frequencies. We call this action "engagement" and "disengagement" of brain frequencies. Our Goal here is to teach you how to better engagement and/or disengage these frequencies to optimize your brain function.

• The Limbic system responses - The limbic part of the brain control all the automatic activities that keep you alive such as; breathing, heart rate blood pressure and much more. We don't have to think about these consciously, which is a good design because consciously we couldn't do it. The limbic system is in constant conversation with the cortex and any pattern of cortical activity that is less than ideal creates challenges in the limbic responses. Our goal is to retrain your limbic responses toward ideal.

• Neurological pattern responses - Over aroused - This is a state where there is too much Beta or not enough Alpha/Theta activity. High cortical activity creates a high demand for glucose (Brain Food). This state puts high demands on the pancreas, liver and adrenal glands. It also keeps the endocrine and immune systems on alert past ideal.

• Neurological pattern responses - Under aroused - A state where there is too little Beta activity or too much Alpha, Theta or Delta. Depression is an outcome of an under aroused nervous system. This state can develop from an over aroused burn out situation.

• Neurological pattern responses - Exhausted - This is a life threatening state of failed neurological function. There has been a break down between the neurological communication and other of the body's systems. The Immune system and the endocrine system no longer respond to the nervous system. Autoimmune diseases are a sign of the body being in this state

• Start with: Chiropractic care to change these neurological patterns - Current research has shown that Chiropractic care has the ability to help your brain reset itself to better balance and engagement. The adjustment stimulates the brain to change and the more appropriate is the adjustment, the better your brain resets toward Ideal function. Retraining the brain takes repetition and training especially when the nervous system has been malfunctioning for years. Along with Chiropractic care, the addition of bio and neurofeedback training will help you achieve better brain function and therefore better overall health.

Stress Response Evaluation Report

Neuro INFINITI

Client: Pre
Session Date: 2/6/2014   Session Time: 12:54:06 PM

Percent Power of EEG

C: EEG (Left)

Theta: Light Sleep-Growth-Repair
Alpha: Focus Learning Meditation

D: EEG (Right)

SMR: Posture-Balance-Readiness
Beta: Busy Brain-High Energy

Heart Rate Variability

Heart Rate

Normative range: 56   to   66   B/min

Skin Conductance

Normative range: 0.80   to   1.50   µS

Temperature

Normative range: 93.92   to   96.98   ° F

Respiration Rate

Normative range: 6   to   12   B/min

SEMG

Normative range: 0.5   to   2.5   µV

A: SEMG (Left)   B: SEMG (Right)

| Eyes Open BL | Eyes Closed BL | Math Test | Recovery 1 |
| Sounds | Recovery 2 | HRV Task | Recovery 3 |

Subjective: Initial: /10   Final: /10   Page   1/2

Stress Response Evaluation Report

Neuro INFINITI

Client: Post
Session Date: 5/5/2014   Session Time: 10:03:14 AM

Percent Power of EEG

C: EEG (Left)   D: EEG (Right)

Theta   Alpha   SMR   Beta   Theta   Alpha   SMR   Beta

Theta: Light Sleep-Growth-Repair
Alpha: Focus Learning Meditation

SMR: Posture-Balance-Readiness
Beta: Busy Brain-High Energy

Heart Rate Variability

Heart Rate
Normative range: 56   to   66   B/min

Very Low   Low   High

Skin Conductance
Normative range: 0.80   to   1.50   µS

Temperature
Normative range: 93.92   to   96.98   ° F

Respiration Rate
Normative range: 6   to   12   B/min

SEMG
Normative range: 0.5   to   2.5   µV

A: SEMG (Left)   B: SEMG (Right)

| ☐ Eyes Open BL | ☐ Eyes Closed BL | ☐ Math Test | ☐ Recovery 1 |
| ☐ Sounds | ☐ Recovery 2 | ☐ HRV Task | ☐ Recovery 3 |

Subjective: Initial: /10   Final: /10   Page   1/2

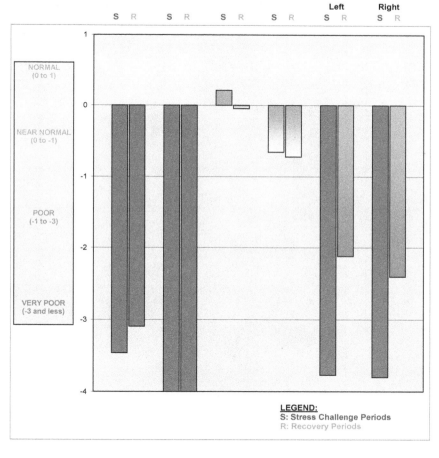

S.R.E. Patient Report

Client: PRe
Session Date: 2/6/2014   Session Time: 12:54:06 PM

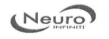

	Heart Rate	Temp.	Resp.	Skin Cond.	Shoulder Muscles	
					Left	Right
	S R	S R	S R	S R	S R	S R

NORMAL (0 to 1)

NEAR NORMAL (0 to -1)

POOR (-1 to -3)

VERY POOR (-3 and less)

LEGEND:
S: Stress Challenge Periods
R: Recovery Periods

Subjective:
Initial: /10
Final: /10

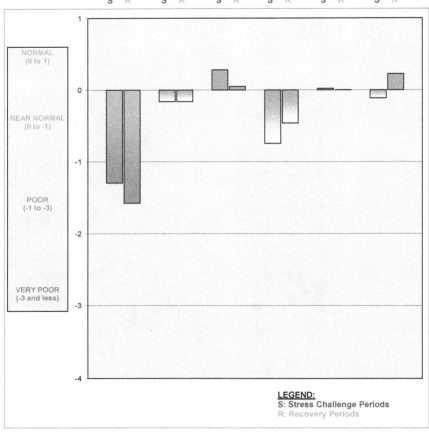

CHAPTER
EIGHT

The High-Tech Solution

Chapter Eight
The High-Tech Solution

Now that we've accurately and thoroughly discussed the problem of stress, the different forms of stress and how people can get trapped in Sympathetic Survival Syndrome; and now that we understand how cortisol and epinephrine levels affect the brain and how it can cause adrenal exhaustion, let's turn our minds to a high-tech solution.

To assist yourself, your family and your friends in dealing with stress, there are only a few things that we know for certain will help the brain get back into harmony, reboot and re-energize. Regular chiropractic adjustments, meditation, deep breathing, deep Delta sleep, exercise and proper nutrition will all help. What you've learned so far is important, but read on. Some revolutionary information is coming. Putting this knowledge to good use will make all the difference in getting great results and living the life you always dreamed you could live NOW.

Biofeedback

Biofeedback is one of the early techniques that came out of research into how we can overcome stress symptoms and keep the brain fit. While that's basically the purpose of this book and the technology it describes, we're not talking about traditional, old-school biofeedback. While there's certainly a place for biofeedback and great results happen over time, the challenge is that it involves the conscious mind, not just the unconscious, which has its limitations. Biofeedback is conducted most often through mind challenges and games. Today, in addition to professional biofeedback therapy, there are several of these games on the market.

Dr. Kaplan developed the dry sensor technology that went into these games, along with neuro-tech guru Paul Donner--who is one of our associates. They created an algorithm that teaches the brain to use brain waves to control or move objects. This is what we mean when we talk about the brain-computer interface. There are many new mind technologies like this being developed on the market. Only recently have we been able to see brain waves as something more than squiggly lines on an EEG machine.

What's amazing is that almost universally the scientists conducting brain research are doing a great job of defining what the problem is, but they are offering few, if any, real solutions to the problem. That's where we come in. We are going to fill that void.

Advancements in technology have allowed us to land on the moon, work from home using computer technology, and have made life much easier to manage. The good news is that this high-tech age has not overlooked emotional health on its path to discovery. State of the art technology has been invented for those people that need a little help to balance their emotional equilibrium.

One such piece of technology utilizes the power of light and sound to facilitate the human mind. No, you read that right. There is a way to harness the power and frequency of these formless entities as you will see when you read on.

Turning on the Lights - A History

Humankind has been using light since the dawn of history. In fact, if you take a trip back in time you'd be sitting in front of the first invented fire, being lulled into a trance like all the other cavemen. Sure, it brought warmth to the cave, but the crackling and flickering of the flames also had a positive, mind-altering effect on the inhabitants.

Attempts have been made to harness the power of light by religious healers and shamans to adopt that half-conscious state. From the light of the sun to a flickering candle flame, what haven't we done to achieve that susceptible state of mind? Our ancestors knew what they were doing, albeit through a different medium, since this state allowed them to create those "spiritual encounters," which we now know were simple hallucinations.

There was a reason for this altered state, though. Gazing into open fires or sunlight allowed them to expand their consciousness, which in turn provided them with innovative ideas that we still enjoy today. Don't confuse this with hallucinations produced as a result of mental illness or the experiences of those unfortunate souls who seek that calming, relaxed state through destructive means such as alcohol or drugs.

Lights, Sound, Action!

Did you know that simple things like the way light strikes your eyes and the way you process sound have the ability to alter your sense of perception? This is because your brain is a receptacle for millions of sensations and images that have accumulated over time. Now, all that information has to go somewhere to prevent overload, right? Many medical doctors studying the brain have found the way to deal with excess information is to have it processed. This is done by stimulating parts of the brain with light and sound technology, which helps de-stress and balance the brain.

Not just any light and sound will do, of course. It takes a certain frequency of both to relax the brain to the extent one can truly feel refreshed. This is where the *Brainwave entrainment* device comes in. This device gives new meaning to the term mind-over-matter. Using state-of-the-art technology, and with extensive research behind its manufacture, the MindFit has the ability to allow you to overcome obstacles you never thought you could. How? Keep reading to find out. You're about to enter a world of SELF-Discovery.

The First Light Machine

Let's take another trip back in time to around 120AD when Ptolemy was working the spinning spoke wheel by placing it between him and the sun. He was the one who discovered the play of light on the eyes caused by this method of spinning the wheel allowed something unique to transpire in the brain--similar to what people using brainwave entrainment experience.

What he actually discovered was that the faster the wheel spokes turned, the brain wave activity increased at the same rate. Chances are, they didn't know what was happening, and you would be wise to stay away from this type of thing if you are unfamiliar with brain wave science or if you are susceptible to seizures.

Marketers and organizations that have nothing more to offer than flickering light machines and very little science behind them are unfortunately pushing untested light technology. On the other hand, there are professionally-designed devices that provide augmented light and sound patterns that have been tested on thousands of clients. For example, Dr. Richard Barwell and his NeuroInfiniti professional team were instrumental in obtaining feedback from users and professionals to help us perfect the brainwave entrainment device.

Coming back to the issue at hand, we have also observed that most people experience a state of well being after experiencing light and sound brain wave training. This is, perhaps, because the brain is the most powerful pharmacy on earth and you have immediate access to it. Imagine what could have been achieved if they had had this technology back in 200AD. What started then has evolved to give us both light and sound as mediums that have extraordinary potential to help us literally rethink our lives and start anew.

What is Self-Mastery Technology?

We are devoted to helping people correct brain stress better, faster and more permanently. Most people are aware that they need to do something. The problem is they have no idea what that something is. They either don't have the tools or they set the bar too high with unrealistic expectations.

Stress is, unfortunately, a part of all our lives. In the 21st Century it has become a more prevalent problem than ever before in human history. What people need to realize is there is no magic potion to get rid of stress completely. Instead, we should be focusing on finding ways to control stress and cope with it more effectively. We need to accept that we will never be stress free, but we can neutralize it and allow ourselves to rebalance and heal more successfully.

The number one thing you need to know about Self-Mastery Technology is that it allows us to change our belief systems. We have to learn that it's not normal to feel lousy all the time. We have to learn to create a new normal; one in which we feel energized, powerful and able to live life to the fullest.

You deserve to be happy, but you can't achieve happiness by inaction. There has to be some change on your part. You also have to be aware that change doesn't happen overnight. It takes work and planning, but change for the better can be achieved. The important thing is to take action every day, no matter how small that action is. Take one action each and every day that will work towards your bigger, long-term goals. Goals can't be achieved by trying something once and quitting. A real, attainable goal is something that is worked on over time.

"I've been using these techniques since I was 12 years old. I learned from my father, who was very much into using self-help strategies. He taught my siblings and I about affirmations and how to visualize and meditate on the

results we wanted to achieve. At first, we primarily used these techniques to achieve outstanding results in sports, but then we discovered that we could apply these principles to any and every part of our lives." ~Patrick Porter

The great thing about your brain is that once you start to use these techniques the brain can generalize into other areas of your life. If we focus our minds on the solutions to the smaller, everyday problems that we face, our brain learns to hardwire itself to deal with the larger problems in the same way.

An Overview of Self-Mastery Technology

Some of you reading this may already be familiar with Self-Mastery Technology (SMT), but for those who aren't, I'm going to give a brief overview. The foundation of SMT is the MindFit light and sound device. When individuals undergo SMT, they simply need to lie back with their eyes closed and the MindFit's precise frequencies of light and sound waves are fed into the brain using specially-designed headphones and glasses. The light pulses are picked up by the optic nerve and even though you can't consciously discern any difference, there is actually a slight frequency difference between the two. It works like binaural beats, or beats using sound, which only 10 percent of the population can discern and respond to.

Light and sound is used in SMT because it models the structure of the brain. The brain uses light and sound to create our space and place in the universe. When we walk into a room, our brain evaluates the light and sound and projects an image of the room. SMT helps us balance the two hemispheres of the brain using the light and sound waves being projected. When the brain begins to synchronize, the body begins to synchronize along with it. The brain is taken from Beta mode and is guided with a very specific algorithm to create a balanced, full-spectrum of brain wave activity.

You might ask, how does the brain know to do that? This is where Dr. Alexander Kaplan's algorithms come into play. We've been studying how the brain responds to light and sound stimulus and what algorithms are needed since the early 80s. In fact, work continues on this today at Moscow State University where Dr. Kaplan, the developer of the SMT algorithms that we use, is the Head of the Human Brain Research Group.

You can even experience this with sounds, where the harmonics can be in the background guiding you from a normal state to a state of relaxation. Once the brain is fully relaxed, it can start to do self-adjustment. Once the body knows what it's like to be in the adjusted state where our innate intelligence tells us that this is the normal function, we can begin to re-educate and reprogram our physiology and neurology to keep it that way.

We have one doctor who uses SMT four to five times a week. He tells us that each time he uses it his experience is different. This is completely normal because the brain is plastic, which means it is always changing. When people listen to SMT, they often sense the light blinking at different intensities. Sometimes they will hear Dr. Porter's voice in their right ear. Sometimes they'll hear it in their left ear. Sometimes they'll hear it in both. Sometimes they'll even perceive having two conversations with them at once. All of this takes place with the sound and harmonics in the background. It all works in harmony to stimulate your brain back into balance.

SMT is truly changing the lives of the people who experience it. We've known people who were afraid of flying and were able to conquer that fear after a few sessions of SMT. Other people had tried unsuccessfully to lose weight for years and were able to lose naturally and effortlessly after experiencing SMT. Even people with insomnia who had resorted to sleeping pills were able to sleep through the night and wake up feeling refreshed and energized after using SMT. The list goes on and on.

SMT is an amazingly powerful tool and it has the added benefit of being completely safe and natural. Our goal with this book is to get more and more people to recognize the benefits it can have in their lives and to start applying the principles they learn towards that goal.

Why Should You Master SMT?

You may be reading this wondering why you should use SMT in your life. If you've ever heard the term, "mind-over-matter," you have your answer. The mind is in control. It is dominant over matter. In this case the matter is our physical bodies. There are immeasurable ways you can improve your physical health simply by changing your mind.

Chiropractors often talk about the concept of above-down and from inside-out. Healing, balancing and maximizing what is above, our brain allows this enormous self-correcting process to take place from above-down and then we express it from inside-out. We are fans of anything that normalizes and maximizes the brain and nervous system functioning and is natural. SMT does this exceedingly well.

It was only a few years ago that scientists were reinforcing the idea that the brain was fixed—that it cannot and does not change. Of course, we now know that this is completely false. In fact, the brain and the nervous system are extremely flexible and always open to change for better or for worse. This incredible ability to change is called neuroplasticity.

Unfortunately, the brain can change for better or for worse. Oftentimes, the stress of everyday life can make the change worse. Through the system we will outline in this book, we know that we can get your brain back to a better, healthier, younger and more vibrant, balanced state, easily and naturally. It's a matter of shifting thinking away from attending to the physical problems in our lives and to that of the mental and emotional as well. It's important to recognize that while pain hurts, stress can kill.

Most people go to a doctor because they're in pain. It's a natural progression that when you feel pain you want to find a way to deal with it and rid yourself of it. That's why we need to recognize that if we want to heal the body, we must heal the brain first. Once the brain is balanced, the body will follow. It doesn't work the other way around.

As I stated before, we've been researching this approach since the 1980s. Dr. Stan Futko, a preeminent chiropractor who has since passed away, was instrumental in bringing the concept of Brain-Based Wellness into the chiropractic clinic. He recognized that when his patients were more relaxed and more at peace, his adjustments were more effective. He operated a Wholeness Clinic at the time--called such because he worked on the whole body—including the brain and mind. We believe today that when someone is stress free, everything works better. To put it another way, "What the brain thinks, the body follows."

You Have Experienced the Benefits of This Phenomenon

Ever been to a movie? You probably don't know this, but the one who invented the moving picture by expanding on the concept of the flickering light on the strobe wheel we discussed earlier was a Belgian scientist by the name of Joseph Plateau. What you experience when you sit in front of the big screen is remarkably similar to that spinning wheel where all this started.

At a certain point, the flickering screen seems to fuse into a steady and un-flickering light pattern, which is what Plateau dubbed "the persistence of vision." Today, this phenomenon allows you to enjoy a movie as your powerful brain assimilates the light pattern as it flows from one scene to another.

The reason we can see a movie, which moves at over 30 frames per second, is because our brains fuse the images and makes them appear as a single moving image. This is how the brain analyzes the useless data and discards it, only presenting what's needed to help solve the current problem you're facing.

This phenomenon didn't end at the turn of the century, though. The French physicist, Pierre Janet, was the one who--while experimenting at a hospital--discovered that flickering lights could be used to reduce hysteria and increase relaxation for patients.

This is exactly how light and sound brainwave entrainment works. Once it trains your brain to think a certain way, it will get you into the appropriate state, which can get you the perfect results that you want. You see, once you master your mind there is almost nothing you can't do.

What if you were told you could have direct access to your unconscious mind using light and sound technology? Boggles the mind, doesn't it?

The year 1990 found me as a researcher using the same technology in Scottsdale, Arizona. We were able to measure the effects of the light strobe through closed eye on the body. Using light and sound experiments, we discovered how these tools actually increased the serotonin and endorphin levels in the brain. These chemicals are responsible for making you feel good. In other words, using precise light frequencies actually allowed us to change a person's body chemistry to produce a large quantity of those neuro-transmitters that can make one feel on top of the world.

The MindFit was observed to demonstrate similar abilities when it was tested on people as well. Imagine your state of mind if you could undergo the mind messaging program to activate the same neuro-transmitters. It would make improving your physical, mental and emotional life a cinch!

And now, this science can be accessed and used by almost anyone on the planet thanks to www.SMTstreaming.com. This technology uses innovative neuro-sensory algorithms in flashing light patterns. It helps train and mold your brain to achieve the most creativity it can get. Your focus and mindfulness also get the attention they need to help you remain alert.

This may seem like a revolutionary idea, but my goal is to see this technology in the hands of every person on earth so that everyone can learn to handle and manage the stress of the 21st Century. This is a science that has seen its fair share of media coverage of late, which I believe will help. In fact, with movies like *What the Bleep Do We Know?* and *The Secret*, more and more people are realizing the power of the mind and how it can be used to overcome the most difficult challenges life can throw at them.

All Light and Sound Machines Aren't Created Equally

This isn't new technology, per se. There have been many therapists and healers across the centuries that have used similar technologies. Anton Mesmer used magnets to cause the "Gaussian Field Effect," that caused the body to feel as though it was asleep or in a deeply relaxed state. This allowed Mesmer to guide his subjects using suggestion. Many people believe that it was the magnets that were responsible for the 'mesmerizing effect,' but I personally believe that it was the suggestions that had people doing Mesmer's bidding. The human mind is actually a very susceptible receptacle of information. It can be capable of making the body do anything with the right suggestions or stimuli. We are capable of astounding feats.

Further on in our timeline, the hypnotists' watch became an iconic symbol of what bringing about altered states was all about. But the watch was only a tool. The hypnotist actually guided the subject to focus on his watch using the rhythm and cadence of his voice and bringing about more relaxed brain wave states. Unfortunately, the swinging watch sometimes gave the impression that hypnotists had some kind of power to bend a subject's mind to his will. However, it was the rhythmic voice and words that that subject was really zeroing in on, not the watch, and the positive altered state achieved is actually a natural, normal response to the right rhythm and cadence, which means the hypnotist's only "power" is that of persuasion.

There are a number of ways to send people into a trance-like state. You can do it with the power of your voice, using simple suggestions or other complex methods. However, successful implementation of most of these techniques takes years to truly master. On the other hand, based on our experiences, we believe the most important element is to get the client out of their limited belief state to place them in a positive, altered state of mind.

What would you say if you found out we can supply you with the brain healing technology using the same methods outlined above? I had the privilege of experiencing this phenomenon firsthand in the 80s while studying the effects of a device called the "Mind Mirror." This device could actually track the user's brainwave activity in real time. The job of the operator was to study the effects of this device by watching a bank of LEDs, while the client was wearing the MC2 light and sound machine.

The results were astounding! Each individual who participated in the three week study was able to demonstrate the level of mind that was programmed into the machine. Once they were able to demonstrate the ability to learn in the Alpha and Theta states, *the sky is the limit with what you can do with this technology.*

The secret to this technology, which is also the point of Brainwave entrainment technology, is to get a person out of Beta, the reactionary mindset. Remember, this state refers to the feelings that are behind one's narrow-minded outlook on life such as fear, anxiety or frustration. As mentioned before, these are the emotions that curb your creative mind and prevent you from making changes. Brainwave entrainment allows the user to overcome or overthrow that debilitating mindset in favor of a positive mentality that then has the ability to help develop a more self-confident personality.

CHAPTER
NINE

**Hebb's Law Helps Explain
Brainwave Entrainment Technology**

Chapter Nine.
Hebb's Law Helps Explain
Brainwave Entrainment Technology

Brainwave entrainment (pronounced: "ehn - TRAIN - mint") refers to the brain's electrical response to rhythmic sensory stimulation, such as pulses of sound or light.

When the brain is given a stimulus, through the ears, eyes or other senses, it emits an electrical charge in response, called a cortical evoked response. These electrical responses travel throughout the brain to become what you see and hear. This activity can be measured using sensitive electrodes attached to the scalp.

When the brain is presented with a rhythmic stimulus, such as a drumbeat or the steady pounding of waves on the beach, the rhythm is reproduced in the brain in the form of electrical impulses. If the rhythm becomes fast and consistent enough, it can start to resemble the natural internal rhythms of the brain, called brainwaves. When this happens, the brain responds by synchronizing its own electrical cycles to the same rhythm. This is commonly called the Frequency Following Response (or FFR)

You've heard us talk a lot about using Brainwave entrainment for various changes you want to make in your life, which is the most advanced brainwave entrainment technology available today. But you may be asking yourself, is there really science behind this theory and does it really work? The answer is a resounding yes and yes! Besides our own decades of experience using this technology and our research into the brain and how it functions, there is sound scientific theory to back up our ideas.

One such scientific principal that has been part of biological and neuropsychological science for over 50 years is Hebb's Law named after Donald Hebb, which states that neurons that fire together wire together. This is a theory in neuroscience, which proposes an explanation for the growth and change of neurons in the brain during the learning process. It describes how the brain's synapses have the ability to strengthen or weaken over time in response to activity or lack of activity. In other words, if you use it--it will get stronger! If you fail to exercise your brain's abilities, it can get weaker--such as in the aging process, while under stress, or when we fall into routines. Our brains are programmed to be able to strengthen, rewire and grow with practice and repetition of skills.

This theory is the basis of neuroplasticity. Neuroplasticity is the way in which our brain reorganizes itself in response to our environment, experiences or injuries. For example, if someone has a stroke and part of the brain tissue is injured, very often the person can still recover the skills lost during the stroke with practice and repetition. Why? Not because the brain heals itself in the particular damaged area, but because the brain can adapt to the new situation and create new neurological pathways. The functions previously performed in that region of the brain are simply shifted to other places on new paths.

This can occur when our brain is made to pay attention such as when learning new skills or practicing skills. When we are learning, we are wiring each experience into our brain's computer for future use. This is basically like exercise for the brain. It causes blood to flow to the prefrontal cortex, which allows hormone release, and hormones protect our brains as we age. Think about it--if you exercise your brain each day utilizing brainwave entrainment, you're not only creating new pathways and strengthening your brain each time, but you're also protecting your brain against the ravages of aging.

Hebbian theory states that repeatedly practicing certain activities can introduce lasting change in our cellular makeup, which adds to the permanency of that cellular make up. However, the best way to do this is to utilize the whole brain. According to Hebb, it's not enough to have, for example, cell A firing alone. Cell A (presynaptic) needs Cell B (postsynaptic) to take up the charge once it's done. What this means is when Cell A continually fires up Cell B, a connection is formed and this bond leads to increases in strength and a new pathway which is the basis for learning and memory. This is what we call whole brain thinking and what we practice when we engage in brainwave training.

One side or the other cannot work alone to cause change. You need both sides to fire together for the most effective learning, thinking and changing possible. Practiced repetition of this, not only strengthens the connection, but also literally increases the size of the connections in the brain to make the changes lasting and permanent. When you utilize MindFit on a consistent basis, these connections can be made and strengthened rapidly and easily.

"The stakes are very high when it comes to letting your brain use you. But if you start to use it instead, the rewards are unlimited." - Super Brain by Deepak Chopra M.D. and Rudolph E. Tanzi, PhD.

Dispelling The Myths

Myth one -

When you injure your brain, such as with a stroke, it can't be healed.

FACT:

Most people would agree, when brain tissue is damaged it doesn't simply grow back the way a broken bone does. What the brain can do, however, is retain skills by creating new pathways in the uninjured parts of the brain to compensate for the parts that no longer function properly. The brain can rewire itself. The way it does this is to exercise and create new pathways to improve memory, thinking ability, behavior, coordination and speech.

According to a study done by the Menzies Research Institute, it was shown conclusively that neurons in the adult brain can remodel themselves away from an injury site and rewire to a different site following injury. This ability provides insight into the brain's huge capacity for plasticity and adaptability. Much research is going into finding the most effective therapies to encourage plasticity in the brain.

We believe brainwave entrainment can be one of these treatments to encourage brain plasticity. We've explained previously how brainwave entrainment encourages whole brain thinking and utilization of brain waves to create change in your life. As you consistently practice exercising your brain, you are actually strengthening and building pathways that will serve you for years to come.

Myth Two-

The brain is static. It's wiring can't be changed.

FACT:

For many generations it was believed that the brain's wiring couldn't be changed. Going back to Hebb's Law, it disproved this myth. This law means that as the brain's cells interact as we learn new things, new circuits are created. In everyday life, if you are learning a new skill, exposing yourself to new experiences, doing things in unfamiliar ways and practicing new skills with repetition, your brain is responding by rewiring itself and strengthening the connections within itself so that as you improve, your brain improves right along with you. We are not hardwired with connections that can't be changed or improved. The brain is plastic, meaning it grows and changes as you grow and change. You have the ability to develop, change and grow in any direction you choose.

Within the last few years what we thought we knew about the brain has completely changed. New testing methods and measuring devices have been invented that can show us maps of the brain and how the brain can change and grow. As recently as 20 years ago, we believed that the mind was static and had a finite number of cells available. Since that time, it's been discovered that the brain is not as fixed and static as previously thought. The brain is plastic, regenerative and trainable.

It's been discovered that as we learn, new neurons are generated in the hippocampus and new pathways are created. The brain is capable of rewiring itself around damaged areas, such as in injury, and can move specific functions to other areas of the brain. Given this information, it wasn't a long leap to realizing that as we repeat any specific brain activity, connections are made and strengthened. The more we practice, the more hardwired that activity becomes--thus creating a default for the brain. If we practice the behaviors that we want, with the use of brain training tools, that new behavior that we desire will become easier and easier until it becomes the brain's natural default action.

According to one study, a research team from Massachusetts General Hospital looked at the brain scans of 16 people before and after they participated in an eight-week course in mindfulness meditation. The results of the study were published in Psychiatry

Research: Neuroimaging concluded that after completing the course in mindfulness meditation, parts of the participants' brains associated with compassion and self-awareness grew while the parts associated with stress shrank.

Sounds a bit like what we've been talking about, doesn't it? Your brain can be rewired for creating new pathways to success, all the while helping you overcome the negative effects that stress has on your life. In other words, you can teach old dogs new tricks.

Myth Three-

As we age we will lose certain brain functions, such as memory.

FACT:

Our goal should always be to live a long, healthy life all the while keeping our brains sharp and focused. Maintaining physical health will mean nothing without a brain that works correctly and in harmony with you. We liken it to a computer--you can have the best hardware in the world, but unless your CPU works properly, it's just taking up space on the desk.

As we age, we have learned to expect that our memories will decline. We'll start to forget little things at first such as where we put our keys or parked our car. As we get older, we believe that those little things can grow into forgetting bigger things. The biggest fear in an aging population is severe mental decline such as in the case of Alzheimer's. In fact, the number one concern of the baby boomer generation is loss of cognitive function.

It doesn't have to be that way, however. The reason the brain ages is because as people age they tend to be less active and perform less strenuous mental activities. The brain is like a muscle. If it's not exercised it can decline.

There are several things you can do to exercise your brain and thus encourage neuroplasticity. These can all help keep your memory and focus sharp no matter what your age.

1.   Exercise. Exercise is one of the single most important things you can do not only for your physical health but your mental health as well. Exercise affects the brain on several fronts. Increased heart rate pumps oxygen to the brain and causes hormonal releases--all of which improve brain function and encourage cell growth. Exercise encourages plasticity in the brain by stimulating growth of connections between cells and creating new neural connections. When you work out to the point that you break a sweat for just 30 minutes per day, your body actually creates new brain cells. How? By increasing the blood flow to your brain and increasing certain proteins supplied to the brain, the hippocampus in the brain actually can increase in size. People with a larger hippocampus are much less likely to develop Alzheimer's.

Exercise is also important because it creates a better attitude and is associated with a drop in stress hormones.   Including yoga in your exercise routine is especially beneficial. Yoga releases tension and stress and allows you to focus on the body and its movements and to "get out of your head" for a while. Yoga also incorporates proper breathing techniques, which allows the body's cells to become oxygenated fully.

2.   Another important factor in brain health is to consciously work on shifting your thinking. Allowing the stress and frustration of daily life to get out of control can actually cause chemical changes in your body which will shrink the hippocampus leading to memory issues.

Learning to relax and release stress is one way to avoid this. Utilizing tools for stress reduction is an ideal way to avoid this issue and reduce stress in your life.

Remaining in the moment is another way to reduce stress. Practicing mindfulness helps us become more aware of our reactions to the stress in the world around us and helps us to slow down from simply reacting--which can increase our stress levels--to being present and choosing our response, which reduces stress because we feel more in control. Mindfulness is a state of active, open attention in the present. When you're mindful, you observe your thoughts and feelings from a distance, without judging them good or bad. Instead of letting your life pass you by, mindfulness means living in the moment and awakening to experience. Mindfulness is that moment in time between stimulus and response where we have time and space to choose a response that doesn't cause additional stress to our brains and bodies.

When you practice creative visualization, for example, you're allowing yourself time to practice mindfulness and be in the moment, reduce stress and practice getting the life you've always dreamed of. All of these things are essential to brain health. Stress reduction reduces the chance of shrinkage of the hippocampus and practicing new skills and techniques encourages the growth of new neural pathways which strengthen your brain and encourages growth--protecting against future aging.

3. Getting proper nutrition to feed your brain will also help decrease the instances of memory issues and brain aging. There's no denying that as we age our body is going to age with us. But getting the best nutrition possible can give your brain the boost it needs to continue to function properly well into your old age.

There are certain "super foods" that can feed your brain the nutrition it needs. Some of these foods include DHA--an omega-3 fatty acid found primarily in fish and supplements. If you get the proper amounts of this fatty acid your hippocampus can increase in size and prevent mental decline. This fatty acid is found in Salmon and other deep water fish, sardines and herring. Because it would be difficult to get a proper amount of omega-3 in our natural diets, supplementation is recommended via fish oils.

Another super food that can feed your brain is blueberries. Blueberries help protect the brain from stress and may reduce the affects of age-related conditions like dementia. Blueberries have some of the highest incidences of antioxidants among all the fruits available in the US. Antioxidants are essential for optimizing health because they combat free radicals that damage cells. This is vitally important to maintaining brain health.

Nuts and seeds are especially important to brain health because they contain vital amounts of Vitamin E. Vitamin E is important because it's an antioxidant but it's fat soluble as opposed to water soluble like other vitamins are. This makes Vitamin E exceedingly valuable in protecting cell membranes, which are fatty as well, by being damaged by free radicals. The brain is very susceptible to damage from free radicals and requires a lot of protection against them. Therefore, taking in adequate amounts of Vitamin E can significantly help prevent cognitive decline as we age. Researchers are studying the effects of Vitamin E intake on preventing serious disorders such as dementia and Alzheimer's.

Avocados are another food that can help keep your brain fit. Avocado is a fatty fruit that contains Omega-3s and Vitamin E, both of which were discussed above. It contributes to a healthy blood flow, which is essential for proper brain function. While avocados are high in calories, they are not empty calories. Avocados contain 20 essential nutrients and vitamins, which makes it one of the best calorie dense foods you can eat.

Dark skinned fruits and vegetables are also recommended to promote brain health. These foods have the highest levels of naturally occurring antioxidants. These foods include kale, spinach, Brussels sprouts, alfalfa sprouts, broccoli, beets, red bell peppers, onions, eggplant, prunes, raisins, berries, plums, oranges, grapes and cherries.

Remember, we don't want you to go too crazy with all these brain foods. Consuming too many calories, no matter the source, can undo all the good effects of these super foods. When you convert glucose to energy, extra oxygen is created and these are the free radicals we spoke about earlier. These free radicals can destroy brain cells. That's why the antioxidants in foods you eat are so important. Brainwave entrainment, used in conjunction with the Self-Mastery Technology audio sessions, encourage you to enjoy a healthy, balanced diet that is best for brain function.

Keeping your brain running at its most effective by fueling it with the right foods. This is one important step to essential brain function as we age. Eating fruits and vegetables in abundance provides the antioxidants your brain needs. Drinking pure fruit juices, such as grape juice can help as well.

Flavonoids are another essential nutrient for brain function. Flavonoids are foods that help protect blood vessels from rupture and protect your cells from oxygen damage. They also prevent excess inflammation in the body. Good sources for flavonoids include apples, apricots, berries, pears, tomatoes and cabbage. They are also found in dark chocolate--so feel free to indulge in a little decadence! In moderation, of course!

4.   Lowering the Big Three. To protect your brain, it is vitally important to do three things: lower your blood pressure, your blood sugar and your amount of belly fat. It has been proven that people who are diagnosed with diabetes have higher instances of Alzheimer's disease. Even people who have elevated blood sugar levels but not the actual diabetes diagnosis are at risk. Allowing your blood pressure to remain high makes your brain slow and sluggish. High levels of belly fat can cause sleep apnea, which leads to brain shrinkage.

Your brain depends on a good blood supply just as well as your heart does to survive. High blood pressure can cause many problems in the brain including stroke, dementia, and mild cognitive impairments. Eating a proper diet and getting exercise are great ways to lower blood pressure. Using brainwave entrainment to reduce your stress and help cement healthier habits in place is another way to help lower your blood pressure.

5.   Always Keep Learning. We have said it previously and we'll continue to say it--the brain is a muscle. You need to exercise it like any other muscle to keep it fit and healthy. As we age it's especially important to continually strive to learn new things and acquire new skills to keep our brains active and sharp and to continually strengthen those pathways. Studies have found that not only does your memory remain intact when you work on new skills, it's improved--and the improvements can last over a long period of time. Mentally challenging activities improve the strength of the pathways in the brain, which strengthens the entire network of the brain. Brainwave entrainment is one way to help exercise your brain. Not only can you rehearse newly acquired skills mentally, but brainwave entrainment also helps with enhanced memory, concentration and focus--all of which create a healthy mind!

6.   Stay Social. And no, we're not talking about Facebook here! It's important to maintain face to face social relationships and interactions as we age. Interacting with people in real world situations requires much more brain power than sitting in front of a computer screen. Communicating with other people in a social setting also encourages the release of endorphins and other good chemicals and reduces excess cortisol in the blood. Cortisol is a chemical that can cause damage and shrinkage to the brain when in excess amounts.

Social interactions also boost brain function because by their very nature they require many behaviors that involve memory, recall and attention. Memory, recall and attention are also required in many cognitive tasks. Strengthening these pathways in the brain through social interaction will assist you as you age.

7.   Breathe! The brain uses three times more oxygen than any other muscles in your body do. That's why it's vitally important for you to breathe completely and deeply and correctly. Your brain is extremely sensitive to oxygen levels and cannot survive long periods of time without the correct levels of oxygen.

To increase oxygen levels in your brain it's important to think about how we physically breathe. We are meant to breathe naturally and without thought through our noses with deep belly breaths. When we breathe normally we move oxygen to the areas of our lungs where the blood circulates. If we don't breathe properly we don't get the proper amounts of oxygenated blood to our brain. Utilizing deep breathing techniques are one way to increase the circulation of oxygen in your blood to ensure the proper amounts of oxygen to our brains. Using brainwave entrainment technology on a regular basis will also help you perfect your deep breathing.

8.   Get Enough Sleep. We spend around a third of our lives asleep, but this time is far from being wasteful. Getting proper amounts of sleep is incredibly important for many aspects of our lives. This is the time when our bodies repair themselves and detox from the previous day. Poor sleep is linked to poor health--both emotional and physical. And while we're asleep our brain is still active and working.

Circadian rhythms regulate all the processes in our bodies from rebuilding cells to digestion. These rhythms are cued by light and dark in our environments and trigger hormone release, body temperatures and other functions. Abnormal rhythms and not getting enough sleep has been linked to obesity, diabetes, depression and even early death, to name a few. When we try to go against our natural circadian rhythms, health problems occur. Even something as simple as staying up late and sleeping late can cause health issues because it interferes with proper hormone secretions and puts unnecessary strain on the body.

Many times we think we can get by on less than the recommended seven or eight hours sleep per night, but this is really not the best idea if you want to continue to maintain your health physically and mentally. Without enough sleep your appetite increases and encourages you to overeat and become overweight. When you don't get enough sleep your body produces less leptin--the hormone that tells you you're full and it produces an overabundance of Ghrelin--which tells you you're hungry, even though you actually aren't.

If you have trouble getting to sleep or maintaining good, deep sleep for long periods of time, brainwave entrainment is an excellent tool to help with this issue. This combination of brainwave entrainment and positive visualization helps in stress reduction, which will help you fall asleep more quickly. It also assists with getting brainwave function normalized to help you not only fall asleep but stay asleep and get better quality sleep.

9.   Get regular chiropractic adjustments. You may be wondering how getting chiropractic adjustments are important to getting and keeping your brain healthy. This was explained in more detail in the chiropractic chapter of this book, but let's just summarize briefly here.

Unfortunately   most   people--including   some   chiropractic professionals--focus simply on chiropractic's ability to relieve pain. Chiropractic provides many wonderful benefits than just that, however. Chiropractic originated for brain and nerve health and its main purpose is to relieve stress on the brain and on the nerves. Chiropractic is the only healthcare profession that focuses solely on improving plasticity in the brain and neurological function.   Chiropractic care, as a regular part of your wellness regime, removes stress and restores normal brain function.

10.   Practice Regular Brainwave Entrainment. As you know from reading this book, brainwave entrainment is the practice of training your brainwaves to fall into step with a stimulus corresponding to a particular brain state--for example Alpha, Theta, Beta, etc--using light and sound in particular patterns. The result of such entrainment is that the brain becomes synchronized causing you to become more optimistic, sleep better, and feel more emotionally stable--among other results. Regular use of your MindFit will help you practice brainwave entrainment and as a result you'll see yourself experiencing the benefits of having a balanced brain almost immediately.

MYTH FOUR -

We lose millions of brain cells every day--and they can't be replaced!

FACT:

While it is true that the brain creates the majority of its cells before we're even born, it's also true that throughout our lives new neurons are created in the hippocampus--the area of the brain where new memories are formed. After these new cells are created, they integrate into the structure of the brain. So throughout our lives, we are creating new cells which can strengthen our brains.

Remember from previous discussions how important the hippocampus is to brain function? As we learn, this area of the brain is strengthened and the foods we eat affect the growth of this area of the brain as well. People who have a larger hippocampus are less likely to have Alzheimer's and other related cognitive issues.

The realization that new brain cells do form throughout life has been an important step in the treatment of Alzheimer's and Parkinson's disease. It may also one day lead to ways doctors can treat brain injuries. For now, however, it's important for you to continue to be able to create these new cells for as long as you can, to maintain brain function. Exercise, proper nutrition and consistently learning new skills are all important factors in making this happen.

As with many parts of our bodies, age does play a role in the production of these new brain cells. As we age, the production decreases naturally. By the time many adults reach the age of 80, they may have lost as much as 20 percent of the neural connections in the brain--leading to decreased memory and recall. It is important, therefore, to continually work to keep the brain active and functioning by use of the above mentioned tools--as well as by utilizing new technologies such as the MindFit. There is no better way to exercise your brain, encourage whole brain function, reduce stress and create new pathways in the brain than by utilizing this technology on a daily basis along with regular chiropractic care.

MYTH FIVE-

The fight-or-flight response will override any other reaction in the brain because we've been genetically coded for generations to react in this way.

FACT-

It is perfectly natural for us to become stressed and anxious from time to time. One of the coping mechanisms that our body uses during these times is the fight-or-flight response. When fight-or-flight is triggered, chemicals such as adrenaline and cortisol are released into the blood stream. Our respiratory rate increases, blood pressure rises, pupils dilate. Fight-or-flight was designed to protect us from physical dangers in our environment. When we faced real dangers in earlier times, this response was very important. However, in society today, other influences such as traffic, arguments, financial instability and relationship issues invoke this response. In this state we tend to see everyone and everything as the enemy. In our super-stressed society, we live life at such a fast pace that we could spend our entire lives in this heightened state. We have lost the ability to relax and allow our bodies to recover from the release of chemicals associated with fight-or-flight.

There is a danger from over-activation of the fight-or-flight response. As we talked about in previous chapters, an overload of these stress hormones can cause disruptions in our lives and bodies and cause a myriad of diseases and conditions that we have to then deal with. We must learn to consciously pay attention to the signals of fight-or-flight and act accordingly to reduce the stressors in our lives. It is possible to rewire the fight-or-flight response and to reduce our reactions to stress in our lives so that the fight- or-flight hormone release does not impact us significantly.

There are several methods we can use to reduce the impact of fight-or-flight on our bodies. We have covered these more in depth throughout the book, but just briefly--remember it's important to exercise to reduce stress, it's important to act in a safe and secure manner and most importantly, it's important to change the way you see the world around you. All of these things can be accomplished through being mindful, and utilizing brainwave entrainment and getting your chiropractic adjustments for stress reduction and relaxation.

In this chapter, we've covered Hebb's Law and the role it plays in the development of your brain. Remember the neurons that fire together wire together. Regular use of brainwave entrainment technology combined with regular chiropractic care is the best defense you'll find against the harmful effects of a stress-filled lifestyle. By regularly guiding your brain into these positive brain states, beneficial change in your life can be made easier and more natural.

Exercising your brain is an important function in keeping sharp and mentally agile through middle age and beyond when most people go into decline. It is possible to keep the brain plastic, changing and growing through adulthood and into our aging years and with Brainwave entrainment as your ally, fear of mental decline can be a thing of the past.

CHAPTER
TEN

All Change Starts in the Mind

Chapter Ten.
All Change Starts in the Mind

Now that you understand the benefits of light and sound technology--also known as brainwave entrainment or audio and visual entrainment (AVE)--it's time to realize how it can change the way the brain works and thus how it can change the way you think.

Let me first introduce you to my dad, Michael J. Porter Sr., who is a genius in his own right. I was 12 years old when he first started training me using a metronome, whose frequency was set to resonate in Alpha (10 cps). Listening to this beat frequency made me adopt an altered state which allowed me to visualize achievement in the sport I was playing.

My father was pretty good at this. He knew, for instance, that he could show me exactly how to use my mind to improve myself in sports and how I could also improve in school. This technique also helped me develop my public speaking skills. The reason my dad was able to do this so effectively was because he was a Silva Method (formerly Silva Mind Control) instructor who had firsthand experience using this technique on others.

He was also very quick to realize how you can actually change a person's awareness and mold their mind into a more receptive state so that they, themselves, could visualize and implement the positive changes they wanted to make in their lives.

Here's how this light and sound technology works for you. The light works on the optic nerve causing it to follow the frequencies being presented, which positively guides the mind into a calmer and more receptive state. The drowsy and comfortable feeling you get is actually a natural byproduct of the brain being gently guided into the Alpha and Theta frequencies.

To put it more simply, your brain will be guided by these beat frequencies causing it to synchronize and organize you into the Alpha and Theta states. This, as mentioned before, will allow your mind, body and brain to harmonize and thus unleash your innate healing powers, benefiting you for a long time to come.

If you're a brainwave entrainment enthusiast, you've probably already heard of binaural beats. Binaurals work by sending one signal into one ear and a different signal into the other ear. For example, if we wanted to create an Alpha state--just one of the frequencies--we could put a 200Hz frequency in the right ear and a 210Hz frequency in the left ear. The brain then, literally, synchronizes the difference, which is 10 cycles, Alpha, because that is the difference between the two.

Unfortunately, this means that binaural beats are not all that effective for people who don't have full hearing range on both sides. The good news is a relatively new brainwave technology called isochronic tones. These tones work on a mono level. So if you don't have full hearing in both ears, it still works for frequency response.

Mind altering technology has been rife in the market and many marketers promote binaural beats to give them a leg up on the competition. However, many of them make claims about efficacy beyond what binaural beats alone can do. Through our research we understand that you can only benefit from these beats if you have the appropriate light and sound technology backing it up.

Why? Without proper synchronization of this technology through a computerized algorhythm, your brain will only be trained to a single brain wave at a time. This just means that your brain can't experience the full effects of the Alpha, Beta and Theta states simultaneously, which comprise a full-spectrum brain wave. When we use both light and sound, on the other hand, it allows the user to experience the full spectrum of brainwaves in each session, thus allowing you to experience Beta, Alpha, Theta and Delta at the same time.

For example, if you were to travel from the UK to the US you would end up crossing several time zones, which puts the body out of balance causing jet lag. Part of this is due to the changes in light frequency but it's also due to the fact that the world is resonating at different frequencies at different places and we tap into those frequencies.

Research has found that our brains and bodies will sync to the frequencies around us. This links with part of the research done by Dr. Kaplan on neuro-acoustic harmonics. His research has shown that we can take certain pieces of music and tune the music so that it is just off-frequency. By doing this we trigger different parts of the brain. This is what brainwave entrainment does. We all know the different parts of the brain control and focus different parts of our personality--as well as memory, concentration and focus, to name a few.

During a brainwave entrainment session, the unit is educating parts of your brain--not with words as we're doing right now--but with different acoustic harmonics. Different harmonics cause the different areas of the brain to respond accordingly. If someone were to take a picture of your brain while you were using the device, you would be able to pinpoint which parts of the brain were affected by which frequencies.

We can also use thermo imaging to see the increased blood flow to various parts of the brain as we trigger and educate those areas. The great thing is that once all this happens, we create the relaxation response. When you're in this pleasurable state, your achievement levels go up and it doesn't feel like work anymore. Once your brain is in balance, it creates a euphoric feeling that keeps you active, energized and better equipped to handle daily stress.

Why Light and Sound Creates the Relaxation Response

As soon as we arrive in the world, we experience the environment around us using our senses and take stock of our world in this way. Your brain is constantly functioning to help you solve problems using whatever environment you happen to be in. With brainwave entrainment, we are using the auditory (sound) and visual (light) senses, engaging the brain's natural ability to sync to the environment.

Picture yourself standing in an elevator and your favorite music is being played. Don't you feel more relaxed and happy than if you weren't hearing it? Don't the lyrics just jump into your mind as soon as you hear the tune? That's because your brain is always searching for solutions to your everyday problems and it uses the rhythm of the words to place those solutions into your psyche. This is how light and sound technology helps us to gain access to the conscious and unconscious levels of your mind.

In other words, brainwave entrainment allows you discretionary access to that part of your brain that has the tools you need to accomplish your goals.

Who Can and Can't Benefit from Brainwave Entrainment Technology?

The majority of the population can benefit from this kind of technology. There are some people, however, who aren't able to use the flashing lights part of this technology but can easily benefit from the sound part of the sessions. If you suffer from epilepsy or seizure disorders like photosensitivity, you should not utilize the lights portion of this technology--or should consult your physician before you do.

Our research, as well as feedback from biofeedback technicians has shown that brighter lights have more chance of providing better results. That's because the more light your optic nerve experiences, the more chances it will have to penetrate the nerve, which in turn increases the chance of activating the brain's neural-network. However, we have also observed in our practice that on average one out of 200 people has some form of light sensitivity and thus prefers dimmer lights. Generally speaking, these are people with light blue or pale green or hazel eyes. Thus, we have a feature on the device that allows the user to choose the light intensity that works best for them.

When the brain is active, it's capable of doing amazing things for you regarding your belief systems. To accomplish this, you have to get to the level of mind that welcomes this sort of change, which is what the Brainwave entrainment can do for you. This technology allows you, the user, to adopt behaviors, attitudes and beliefs that can literally give you a new lease on life!

Does the Music Really Matter?

For most of us, learning means absorbing as much information as we can--either in a classroom setting, within a social gathering or just from interacting with the environment. In fact, learning is so ingrained, we do it on an unconscious level in stressful situations so that we can find solutions to get out of those circumstances. Because so much of what we learn is through the unconscious mind, most of us remember only a small portion of what we've actually absorbed.

Wouldn't it be great if you could make your learning experience more efficient in an environment that facilitates optimum brain power so you never have to search your memory for information again? The good news is this type of learning is possible via a technique called accelerated or super learning. This method consists of a set of innovative techniques designed to specifically help one assimilate knowledge faster and with regularity. One of these methods uses the power of sound or music to help people strengthen their mental processes.

This process basically refers to the association between a specific stimulus and a state of mind, feeling, idea or thought. The famous Russian physiologist, Ivan Pavlov, was the first to discover this phenomenon in his dog experiment, which we discussed earlier. Why did this work? Hearing the bell for extended periods allowed a neurological link between the dog's hunger and the bell. That's called an anchor.

This technique is often used to create an associative state between the stimulus and the neurological system of the human mind so that the resultant action seems natural or automatic on the part of the subject.

Now, you're probably wondering what does music--a form of entertainment for most people--have to do with super learning? Actually, it has a lot to do with it. As mentioned before, your mind has the ability to function in different brain wave states.

Remember, Alpha is the state that is crucial for learning to take place. Some Theta waves also come into the equation during this period--between the highest Theta waves and the lowest Alpha waves-- so that positive ideas are generated.

The famous otolaryngologist, Alfred Tomatis, was the one who discovered that the design of the ear not only aids the hearing process but also acts as a natural energizer for the brain and body. Tomatis gleaned the result from studying various pieces of musical compositions by Bach, Mozart and the Gregorian chants.

Tomatis discovered that the above-mentioned pieces had high

frequencies that actually had the ability to charge brain cells and release muscle tension. Remember the shamans and "psychic" healers? Their psychic abilities come from the state of mind they experienced when they went into trances. Since their mind was more open to suggestions, it made them susceptible to all supernatural experiences.

You can probably understand by now why music is such a big deal with this type of technology. That's why we regularly utilize music and tones so that your brain can achieve the proper state for super learning to take place.

Think about it. When you're at the movies, the music plays a crucial role in the development of the story--whether you're consciously aware of it or not. Composers and musicians have grasped and developed this idea so that more and more people could share in the transcendent experience during a show. They understand how specific rhythms and tones and sounds of music they play have the ability to influence the mood of the audience. Does it work? How many movies have you enjoyed that have no soundtrack working behind it?

At PorterVision, we've incorporated these ideas into our systems by playing soothing music during our audio sessions. We have discovered that the brain can actually move into the Alpha state when the subject is listening to Baroque style music, which as we mentioned before, refers to a heightened level of awareness, intuitiveness and concentration. When this improves, it automatically accelerates your thinking process and comprehensive abilities, causing accelerated learning.

What's That Sound? Binaural Beats

Now that we've shown you how this technology can benefit you, it's time to discuss what tones have to do with the entire equation. These are the components that actually induce relaxation.

To talk about binaural beats, we'll have to travel back in time again to 1839 where an associate professor at the University of Berlin named Dove discovered that if a person is made to hear different frequencies in each ear, he or she can actually hear a third frequency. This extra frequency had the ability to synchronize the brain of a listener into specific mindsets, like Alpha, to guide them into a state of awareness.

These are called binaural beats. They are produced when the brain combines the separate tones and makes a single tone. The single tone pulses according to the brain frequency you prefer, thus creating the perfect, relaxed state for you. Once the central nervous processor relaxes as it synchronizes with the frequency that generates a natural reaction from it, it causes your body to follow suit. Incidentally, this experience is exactly what you get when you use brainwave entrainment technology in combination with a Self-Mastery Technology audio session.

Let's say we want to create the Alpha brain wave state at 10Hz frequency. To do that we'd place 190Hz frequency in one ear and 200Hz in the other. The subject's brain will synchronize to produce the 10Hz, the difference between the two frequencies, and begin to function in the Alpha state. In this state you can visualize your desires and gain the confidence you need to realize your goals in real life.

This ideal state of mind is achievable with brainwave entrainment technology. Through modern science and this light and sound technology, everyone can experience the deep states of Theta that are necessary for weight loss, pain-free childbirth, stress reduction, sports enhancement, or kicking the smoking habit. These are just a few of the amazing programs available at www.self-masterytechnology.com.

That's not the end of the research, though. In 1960, Andrew Near discovered how EEG patterns of a person changed with rhythmic and natural pounding of a drum. That's what the shamans were able to do. Through the rhythm and cadence of natural drum beats, they had the ability to put the whole tribe into a trance-like state to make them more susceptible to healing experiences. This expanded state of consciousness has always been sought by healers, shamans and life coaches so that the spiritual experience might open the doors to new beginnings in our lives.

A World Full of Experts

The World Wide Web may have given us greater access to help for various issues, but it has also been responsible for putting forth questionable "experts" in the field of mind technology. Check out Apple Store or Google Play apps and you'll find a number of featured binaural beats that claim to do everything from getting you back your lover, bringing you untold riches, or giving you the slim body of your dreams.

Those dreams can only become a reality if you use the correct and scientifically-tested methods that boost your brain power. Why? There is no science that shows being in a certain brainwave state creates anything but that brainwave state. Say good-bye to the app that promises to woo your sweetheart back to you or line your pocketbook. It just doesn't work that way.

What you're actually seeing out in the world is the way all those different binaural technologies train the brain to create a singular brain wave. What the brain does best is habituate, so once you've listened to one of these audios a few times, the brain just follows the same neuro-pathway as before, and all brain fitness benefits are lost. The binaural beats do have the power to make your mind follow that frequency into an altered state (assuming you have balanced hearing), but there's little long-term benefit to it.

We do things differently. We help people realize that brain balance and the power of positive thinking are the only things that can permanently help them, which is why we've taught more than 900 chiropractors to use this Brain-Based Wellness approach, and with dramatic results.

This is also why we've developed an entire library of audio-recordings for those people who want to upgrade their thinking prowess while achieving brain balance. We have used and become experts in the field related to language patterns for this very reason. Our sessions provide you with the motivational thoughts that trigger the highly receptive Alpha and Theta brainwaves. This is where you can pick from over 500 messaging systems to find one that is in accordance with your improvement level.

As mentioned before, your brain is constantly listening to and observing the world around you and adapting accordingly. This is a process known as the reticular activating system. Have you ever felt like dancing when you were at a party, even though you weren't particularly interested in being there? That happens because your brain is trying to adapt to the environment it finds itself in based on past experiences that are in sync with it.

You can't tell it's happening, but your brain is always actively searching for hidden dangers as well. It will be searching for past experiences that can help it identify the current situation you're in to make you feel more comfortable and at ease. In fact, this biofeedback mechanism is why you feel comfortable with people you perceive as being like you and can't wait to get away from people with conflicting beliefs or lifestyles.

We have also observed this phenomenon when interviewing people who used our technology by playing specific music while speaking with them. By listening to Alexander licensed music during the interview, we found people were more open to share their experiences with brainwave entrainment than they were if the music wasn't playing.

All this technology requires is that you don the LED glasses and your favorite earphones and allow the NeuroSensory Algorithms (NSA), which we'll explain later, to guide you through the brain fitness process. You will experience the deep relaxation needed to achieve your goals in peace and harmony without having to do more than close your eyes, take a deep breath in and relax.

What About Isochronic Tones?

The latest brainwave entrainment technology, Isochronic tones, are manually created equal intensity pulses of sound separated by silent intervals. They turn off and on in rapid succession according to the brain frequency needed and are particularly easy for the brain to follow.

Light Frequencies...for Your Eyes Only?

Most people think we only perceive light through our eyes, but nothing could be further from the truth. You see, light is made up of vibration, as is almost everything else in our world, and our lives depend on this symphony of vibrations.

This vibrational symphony frequencies is our universal language. Every form of life is made up of and depends on frequencies. In other words, we are actually comprised of light and sound. The light we see and the sounds we hear are in the visible and auditory vibratory ranges, but there are countless others that vibrate faster and slower than those we see or hear.

The Earth itself has its own magnetic frequency field. We are always immersed in this invisible frequency field. The Earth frequency varies within a limited range, with 7.83 Hz considered the base frequency, which today is known as the Schumann Frequency, named after the scientist who discovered it.

Our external and internal environments are continually affecting the vibration of our cells. Thoughts, emotions and words, whether beneficial or harmful, directly influence these vibrations, just as what we think and say influences our brain wave activity. Nutrition and environmental issues such as air pollution also affect the vibration of our cells.

If vibrations are not in a healthy range for our cells, the seeds for diseases are sown. These disease-causing or toxic vibrations allow pathogens such as viruses, bacteria, fungi and molds to grow.

Vibrations are measured by frequencies called Hertz (Hz) relative to the number of times an object vibrates in one second. This is also referred to as cycles per second.

For example, the power that operates our household appliances is delivered at a frequency of 60 Hz in North America and 50 Hz in Europe.

For decades, many experts have warned that these speeds of vibration that power our household appliances are having an unhealthy effect on us and are adding to our toxic burden. And now, with the plethora of electronic devices in our world, we experience a 24/7 barrage of frequencies that don't support the health of our cells. For this reason, tools that expose the body's cells to healthy frequencies can provide countless benefits.

This is the driving force behind the resurgence of energy medicine, which works to restore the body's natural frequencies or vibrations to improve health. It is the foundation of most alternative medicine practices such as chiropractic (which we already discussed), homeopathy, acupuncture, and Reiki to name a few.

Acclaimed French neurologist, Dr. Paul Nogier, through meticulous research with the subtle energies of the body, made an amazing discovery—he charted three frequencies that stimulate the creation of our bodily tissues:

1.   Tissue known medically as the ectoderm, including outermost tissue that forms skin, glands, nerves, eyes, ears, teeth, brain and spinal cord.

2.   Tissue known medically as the endoderm, including innermost tissue that forms the lining of the intestinal tract, lungs, bladder, urethra and auditory tube.

3.   Tissue known medically as the mesoderm, including middle tissue that forms connective tissue, heart, blood and lymph vessels, kidneys, ovaries, testes, spleen and cortex of the adrenal gland.

In total, Nogier classified seven frequencies natural to our bodies— three frequencies that correspond to these three tissue types plus four additional frequencies.

His research shows that the application of these frequencies helps to bring organs and tissues back to their healthy resonant frequency. A resonant frequency means the natural frequency with which an object, in this case the body's cells, vibrates.

Cells are considered to have the ability to pick up their particular resonant frequency when they are exposed to a range of frequencies that includes their particular natural healthy frequency.

Nogier famously used the ear meridians to deliver these healthy frequencies, which include a full octave of sound, color and light, with astounding results.

Today, energy medicine is a term well-known in the realm of natural health, but just now is coming into public awareness thanks to medical pioneers such as Dr. Mehmet Oz who stated, "As we get better at understanding how little we know about the body, we begin to realize that the next big frontier in medicine is Energy Medicine."

Other medical experts are recognizing the validity of energy medicine and acknowledging its historical relevance, including visionaries such as Albert Szent-Györgyi, Nobel Laureate in Medicine, who acknowledged, "In every culture and in every medical tradition before ours, healing was accomplished by moving energy."

When we apply healthy frequencies through light and/or sound, our cells have the opportunity to absorb the frequencies with which they naturally vibrate to keep us healthy. This is the purpose of the Nogier frequencies.

In relation to the MindFit, the newest and most advanced brainwave entrainment technology to date, we've included the Nogier frequency known for it's ability to create a strong parasympathetic response, helping to calm the nervous system and relax muscles. Like Dr. Nogier, we deliver the light frequency through the ear meridians rather than through the optic nerve. This form of light therapy is known as auriculotherapy.

To accomplish this, we strategically placed 9 medical-grade LED lights in each of the earphones. In doing so, we've found that even those experiencing brainwave entrainment for the first time can generate and sustain the equivalent Theta brain wave activity to those who had consistently meditated for more than 15 years. Keep in mind that without disciplined meditative practice, Theta is very difficult to sustain for more than a few moments at a time.

We also saw even more improvement in overall function of the regulatory systems of the body when we used the HeartQuest HRV before and after 20-minute brainwave entrainment sessions that included auriculotherapy.

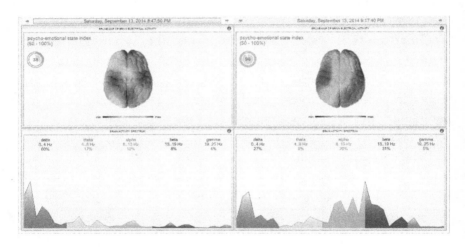

In the HeartQuest Panel above you can see how Randy, an 82-year old retired psychologist, went from a 34 psycho-emotional state to a 96 in just one session with the new MindFit technology.

CHAPTER
ELEVEEN
The Research that
Will Blow You Away

Chapter Eleveen.

The Research that Will Blow You Away

Now, after reading all that, do you realize how much time and effort has gone into producing the best technology to achieve the best results? It's real and it has huge implications for the way we think and act in our everyday lives.

We had the privilege of watching the effects of this technology firsthand when the Pain-Free Lifestyle series was part of an in-house study done at the American Pain and Wellness Clinic in Plano, Texas. They discovered that by using light and sound technology, they could alleviate the pain of those patients that weren't able to find relief through drugs or surgery.

This was a 12-week study where each of the 30 participants was given their own brainwave entrainment technology to use at home once a day--up to three times per day if they wanted to and were able. Dr. Remer and Dr. White tracked the subjects, observing that each subject was able to tolerate pain better. Thirty-five percent of the test subjects felt no pain whatsoever, and another 35 percent reported a considerable reduction in their pain levels after the brainwave entrainment session.

You have to keep in mind that this was possible using light, sound and strategic mind messaging sessions. This is a natural process. The brain is the most powerful pharmacy on earth. Imagine what it could do for you today just by allowing the natural processes of your mind do what it does best--making your life a whole lot easier to live.

You can imagine our joy when Dr. Remer called us and asked whether it was normal for the subjects to lose weight while using the device. Apparently the average weight loss experienced was just under a pound a week--and all with no mention of weight loss within the sessions the subjects listened to. This happened because naturally fat burning hormones are activated when the body undergoes a deeply relaxed state.

In this state, cortisol levels are normalized, thus speeding up the fat burning rate during the process. This phenomenon could also have been the result of a psychosomatic release as well, which compelled the patient to create the weight as a buffer against the pain. The deep relaxation effect of the device had allowed them to negate or eradicate the pain they felt, reducing the stress response, and thus eliminating the resultant weight as well.

Later in the chapter you'll learn about other doctors who conducted breakthrough research in which they measured the subjects' blood levels before and after they went through the light and sound therapy sessions. They observed an average increase of endorphin levels at 25 percent and 21 percent for serotonin levels, which led them to conclude that photic stimulation is one of the greatest breakthroughs ever discovered when it comes to decreasing depression and other related symptoms.

That's great news for you! Thanks to advancements in technology, you can now have the privilege of owning your own brainwave entrainment device that can literally mold your mind into a mechanism designed to make you feel good all the time.

The Secret Sauce

A woman once walked up to renowned painter, Vincent Van Gough, and asked him to sketch her portrait in charcoal. The artist complied and drew the perfect portrait and handed it to her. Pleased, the woman asked how much she owed him; to which he replied, "$700." When she asked why he was charging such an astronomical sum for a simple charcoal sketch that only took a few minutes to make, the artist replied that it had actually taken his whole life, not just the few minutes she saw.

The MindFit has also been honed and perfected using a similar timeframe. We and other researchers have worked thousands and thousands of hours in Neuro-Sensory Algorithm sessions to make sure that this technology delivers the best results possible. Dr. Richard Bandler, Dr. Paul Donner and myself have made sure that the MindFit brainwave entrainment device meets all the requirements individuals need to relax and let go of all their worries.

Between our group of researchers, business partners and field therapists and us, we believe it's safe to say that that no other organization can boast the level of field testing or user feedback that we have completed.

That being said, let's go back to our discussion of how Beta, Alpha, Theta and Delta brainwaves determine your state of mind according to their fluctuation levels. Those four frequencies are basically the "secret sauce" that powers brainwave entrainment. How? Let's expand on that.

As mentioned before, Beta waves are those that set you in the reactionary state of mind. The stimulus that occurs in this state of awareness has to be transferred in the other-than-conscious part of your brain so that it shows up in the form of new behavioral patterns upon awakening. This is difficult to accomplish from the Beta state.

We have ingrained within us what psychologists call the critical factor, which is a part of the mind that is continually relating and comparing new information to what we already know. It's a great system for helping us identify the world around us, but for many it can also set fixed patterns based on what we've previously experienced. We know these as opinions, beliefs and habits, and they can discourage change from taking place.

We have found a way to bypass this reactionary mindset and move from Beta into the Alpha and Theta mindsets. Why? As you know by now, Alpha brainwaves are those that rely on intuitive knowledge that the mind generates.

In other words, this is the part of your psyche that knows what you have to do to improve your life; however, most people have difficulty letting this brainwave work for them because they haven't used it enough. We have to bring those waves to a deeper state or Theta level to engage the inventive mind.

This state is where you have breakthrough dreams and eureka moments that characterize inspiration. Incidentally, this is where pain-free childbirth and surgery are possible.

This is the state you want to engage as part of the full-spectrum brain wave activity we've discussed. However, who has the time to take a break from life and trek to the highest mountain for a session with a Zen master?

This is why for more than sixty years scientists have studied brain wave activity, looking for ways to get the same benefit in less time and with little effort. Today, in twenty minutes or less, the average person can achieve the same optimized brain states that it would take Zen masters fifteen or twenty years to accomplish.

How Brainwave Entrainment Affects the Stages of Sleep

Are you one of those individuals who has to go one-on-one with the sheets before you can drift off into an exhausted stupor? Don't worry. You're not alone. Millions of people suffer the same frustrating ritual once the sun calls it a day.

One of the most harmful misconceptions that people have today is that the body just turns off for several hours and turns back on when it's time to get up. That's simply not true. Believe it or not, the sleep state is an active state, since brain activity is at its most varied at this time.

Without the proper use of light, sound and the appropriate algorithm to make them work, our brains will simply bypass the Theta state and go to sleep. But with the right brainwave entrainment tool, this doesn't happen. Anyone can experience the extensive healing state this device can generate if they want to recharge their batteries, relax or just take a quick nap.

Unfortunately, many people believe that Delta refers to a state of mind that aids sleep-learning. There is no learning experience happening there. Why? Your brain is actually functioning between 0-4Hz at that time, a frequency that discourages learning from taking place. That doesn't mean your mind is sitting idle. This kind of deep sleep is necessary for the brain and body to rejuvenate, which is only possible if one is in deep, Delta sleep. This is good news for those who experience frequent bouts of schizophrenia, depression, anxiety or other negative emotional states.

You see, as soon as your head hits the pillow, you have actually moved through each of the brain wave frequencies. First, you start off predominately in Beta, which is an alert state, one that you can experience when you're having trouble dozing off. This is the reactionary mind, which can be curbed and greatly benefits from brainwave entrainment, which moves you from Beta to Alpha and Theta so that you drift off naturally into a full and relaxed sleep.

This is the feedback we've received from thousands of clients we have used this technology. Most of them are happy to report to us that they haven't experienced a sleepless night after they started regular brainwave entrainment. Many even say using the device for twenty minutes during the day makes them feel as though they've had a three or four hour power nap.

The reason people feel so rejuvenated after using brainwave

entrainment technology is because we're able to make them experience the effects of deep sleep, which, as any neuro-scientist will tell you, is responsible for the release of growth hormones and reduced protein breakdown in the body. Reduced activity is also observed in those parts of the brain that control emotions, aid decision making and influence social skills.

This suggests that the type of sleep you get can help you maintain favorable emotional and social functioning while awake. This has also been determined in a study of rats, which revealed that rats were prone to generate certain nerve patterns throughout the day. This is the repetitive pattern that helps to encode memories and thus aids in the learning process.

It's hard to believe, but it's true. When a subject wears our technology, his or her brain undergoes an exercise regime that makes brainwaves switch from Beta to Alpha and Theta. It then proceeds to dip ever so subtly into Delta, or deep sleep state, which is why people feel so rejuvenated when they complete a session.

How is that possible? Because we have found a way to make you feel as though time were suspended, when it's actually not. You see, when you enter into the space that characterizes the interval between the brain fitness session and Alpha, Theta or Delta brainwaves, time seems to stop.

This is the state one gets into when one sees a picturesque landscape or an attractive member of the opposite sex. On the opposite end of this spectrum, doesn't time seem to crawl when you're experiencing something distasteful?

The reason this strange phenomenon occurs, is because the thoughts generated during the experience tend to change, making the frequency respond accordingly, thus altering the perception of time. When you dip into Alpha and Theta this way, you tend to experience expanded time periods, which you can use as an expanded timeline to improve the quality of your life in a matter of minutes. All of this happens at the other-than-conscious level of your mind, resulting in complete relaxation.

Your Brain Doesn't Know
the Difference Between Real and Imaginary

How does that happen? Because your brain is not structured to decipher what's real and what's not. This is why we use spoken word guided visualizations, guiding the mind to replace negative thoughts with more creative and positive ones. These are then incorporated into the learning process and can be played back via the behavioral changes that can make the difference you want in your life.

Why are such drastic measures necessary? Making changes in your life isn't easy, especially if you have to rethink everything you've ever believed to make the change. However, this is the level of mind/brain modification required if you want to rebuild yourself from the ground up. Light and sound technology does the same thing by exposing you to information you've never seen, heard or experienced before.

Those of you who might have experienced this phenomenon before by either reading about it or physically experiencing it are at a state of "conscious incompetence." You have some knowledge but not the vast amount that we've accumulated since the '80s while studying this subject. Once you've read this whole book and are able to use this technology, you'll reach the level of "conscious competency" and be given the opportunity to continue your personal transformation.

What Does the Research Say About Brain Chemistry?

It's important to note that up to 100 percent of excess adrenaline is flushed from the system every time the relaxation response is achieved-

-which is the opposite of the fight-or-flight response. This alone is a dramatic result considering that over-production and retention of adrenaline is one of the most dangerous effects of stress on the body because it adds an unnecessary toxic burden on the body.

One of the most important neuro-chemicals released during a brainwave entrainment session is norepinephrine, the hormone and neurotransmitter most responsible for vigilant concentration. Research shows an 11 percent rise in a user's level of norepinephrine after just one session of brainwave entrainment.

Additionally, the same research shows that serotonin levels increase by 21 percent on average. This helps the brain eliminate excess stress chemicals, which is, of course, the desired outcome.

Most people don't realize that nearly 90 percent of the human body's total serotonin is located in the gastrointestinal tract, where it is used to regulate intestinal movement. The remainder is synthesized into the serotonin neurotransmitter, which has various functions including the regulation of mood, appetite, and sleep, and is widely believed to be the neurotransmitter that affords feelings of contentment, wellbeing and happiness. Serotonin also plays a role in cognitive function, including memory and learning.

Serotonin is normally utilized by the brain and then flushed out. This is one of the major concerns about many anti-depressant medications, which are designed to keep serotonin in the brain longer. It can be likened to keeping food in your refrigerator longer with the hope that it will somehow become more nutritious.

In the same way, storing serotonin in the brain is not likely to help the brain work better—and keeping old serotonin in the brain can have unknown damaging effects—because this is not how serotonin works in the brain.

Used serotonin needs to be flushed out to allow the brain to create new neurochemicals and restore balance. The brain knows how to create these balanced pain-free states naturally, it just needs the opportunity to do so, which is where the relaxation response comes into play.

Chemical reactions occur in the body based on the brain wave state we're currently in, which is directly linked to our thoughts and perceptions at any given time.

When we're trapped in a high Beta mode, we don't have the Alpha and Theta patterns to tell the brain to create the new neurochemicals that make us feel balanced and content because it's stuck in fight-or-flight mode. We need to take action to ensure that the sympathetic system is able to relax and interact with life instead of reacting to life. When this happens, the brain is bathed in all the positive neuro-chemicals it needs for balance and a healthy outlook on life, and there is no need for medication.

In a study performed by the Shealy Institute of Comprehensive Health Care in Springfield, Missouri, in 1990 with Dr. Roger K. Cady and Dr. Norman Shealy called, "Neurochemical Responses to Cranial Electrical Stimulation and Photo-Stimulation via Brain Wave Synchronization," (11pp), 11 patients had peridural and blood analysis performed before and after relaxation session using flash emitting goggles. An average increase of Beta-endorphin levels of 25 percent and serotonin levels of 21 percent were registered. The Beta-endorphin levels are comparable to those obtained by cranial electrical stimulation (CES). This study indicates a potential decrease of depression related symptoms when using photic stimulation.

Additionally, beta-endorphins are more potent pain relievers than morphine, which is why so many people report pain relief as a natural side effect of a brainwave entrainment session that includes Alpha and Theta training.

What Does the Research Say About Visualization?

In a study published in Psychology and Health, 177 students were asked to set the goal of consuming more fruit. All the students ended up eating more fruit, but those who visualized how they were going to carry it out increased their fruit consumption twice as much as those who didn't use visualization.

Many of the visualization techniques used in SMT are borrowed from sports psychology. According to one researcher, "Athletes do lots of work mentally rehearsing their performances before competing and it's often very successful. So we thought having people mentally rehearse how they were going to buy and eat their fruit should make it more likely that they would actually do it. And this is exactly what happened."

What if you could double your motivation to accomplish your goals? What might you achieve?

In another study that related visualization to binge eating, researchers used similar guided imagery techniques to those used in SMT. The imagery group had a mean 74 percent reduction in bingeing. The imagery treatment also demonstrated improvement on measures of attitude concerning eating, dieting and body weight in comparison to the control group.

Another one of the great things about Self-Mastery Technology versus other methods of dealing with stress is that there are no negative side effects. We tell our clients that the only possible side effect you may experience while using this technology is that you could fall asleep, have a good nap and wake up with a life changed for the better.

The only contraindication to using SMT technology would be that flashing lights are not recommended for people who have epilepsy or other seizure disorders. These people are able to listen to the audio portion of the programs, but we eliminate the light portion. Fortunately, those people are still able to get excellent results with SMT because the light frequency is only one of five technologies designed to work together in the SMT algorithms.

Whether your aim is to improve your learning, balance your brainwaves, normalize blood pressure, improve your energy, lift your mood, eliminate addictions, become healthier and happier or become more assertive, you will find that all of these can be side benefits of SMT. Remember when the brain is in balance, the body will follow and we call this healing.

We know through research that when the neurons in the brain start firing together they also start wiring together. This means that we're actually teaching the brain to wire itself to achieve new levels of efficiency and the brain loves that. The brain is a like a muscle. It is designed to be used and the more it's used the better it performs. We've had dozens of open and real-time live sessions in which we've tracked the brain waves from the patient's wide awake state into the relaxation response. Like clockwork, we see the Beta brain waves come down as Alpha and Theta go up--until balance is achieved.

Conversely, if the brain is sedentary, such as passively watching television, it begins to lose the new levels of wiring that you have worked hard to create. This is why websites like Lumosity have become so popular. The brain wants to be functioning and used and a brain game is one way to make this happen. SMT is another way--a fun, relaxing way to take a power nap, giving the brain its neurological exercise.

We'd like to just briefly share with you an experience that we had at a training with our affiliate, Dr. Richard Barwell, and his team. Dr. Barwell hooked up one of the doctors at the training to his NeuroInfiniti biofeedback system, which utilizes EEG to view brain wave activity. We all watched the results on a TV screen, which clearly demonstrated that his brain waves were out of balance. When the demonstration began, we could all clearly see how his sympathetic and parasympathetic systems were firing at completely different rates.

We then placed this doctor on a Self-Mastery Technology session. Remarkably, after six or seven minutes on this technology, we could see on the TV screen how the brain came back into balance and harmony. The sympathetic and parasympathetic systems were soon firing equally. It was a jaw-dropping experience for most of the people in that room-- to visually see a demonstration of how this technology really can bring the brain back to balance and harmony.

There is a lot of research suggesting that simply taking a mid-day nap can be very beneficial. We jokingly say that SMT is like taking a nap on steroids. It helps stimulate the process of flushing out the excess cortisol and adrenaline from your system, stimulating healthy neurochemistry as outlined in the Shealy Institute research study on neurochemical response, and bringing the system back into balance, much in the same way you do when you achieve deep, Delta sleep at night.

References:

Dr. Roger K. Cady, Dr. Norman Shealy in "Neurochemical Responses to Cranial Electrical Stimulation and Photo-Stimulation via Brain Wave Synchronization." Study performed by the Shealy Institute of Comprehensive Health Care, Springfield, Missouri, 1990, 11 pp.:

Fruitful plans: Adding targeted mental imagery to implementation intentions increases fruit consumption. Barbel Knauper, Amanda McCollam, Ariel Rosen-Brown, Julien Lacaille, Evan Kelso, Michelle Roseman. Psychology & Health, 2011

A randomized controlled trial of guided imagery in bulimia nervosa.

Esplen MJ1, Garfinkel PE, Olmsted M, Gallop RM, Kennedy S. Psychol Med. 1998 Nov;28(6):1347-57.

Direct Effects of Audio-Visual Stimulation on EEG
M. Teplan, A.Krakovska, S. Stolc

Stress Reduction by Technology? An Experimental Study into the Effects of Brain Machines on Burnout and State Anxiety
Dr. Hans C Ossebaard

The Comorbidity of Eating Disorders and Attention Deficit Hyperactivity Disorder
Sharon K Farber PhD

Brain Wave Synchronizers; A Review of Their Stress Reduction Effects and the Clinical Studies assessed by Questionnaire, Galvanic Skin Resistance, Pulse Rate, Saliva, and Electroencephalograph
Donald R Morse DDS,MA(Biol), MA(Psychol), PhD(Nutr)

A Comprehensive Review of the Psychological Effects of Brainwave Entrainment
Tina L. Huang PhD, Christine Charyton PhD.

Symposium Looks at Therepeutic Benefits of Musical Rhythm
Emily Saarman; Stanford News Service

A Study of Brainwave Entrainment Based on EEG Brain Dynamics
Tianbao Zhuang, Hong Zhao, Zheng Tang; Computer and Information Science

C H A P T E R
TWELVE
Technology for Our Time

Chapter Twelve.

Technology for Our Time

Let's go back for a moment to when my dad, Dr. Michael J. Porter, Sr., and I first set out to use light and sound technology in what later became our franchise company. My father is one of those people who believe "old school" never goes out of style, which is why he was quick to be doubtful about the benefits of brain wave entrainment technology. His argument was, "Why use a device when I can do all of those on my own, using my voice and the process of visualization?" My dad wasn't someone you wanted to argue with once he got his teeth into an idea.

It was the '80s, back when smoking was still considered cool. Fifty-five percent of Americans smoked but many of that 55 percent wanted to quit the habit. This compelled us to open a chain of stop-smoking clinics with our associate, Dr. Paul Adams, now deceased, (who opened three clinics in Detroit). My dad opened a clinic on the west side of Phoenix and I opened up in a chiropractic clinic on the east side and in Scottsdale, Arizona.

Our clinics were each a bit different. We had all gone through getting our master practitioner license in Neuro-Linguistic Programming with its co-founder, Dr. Richard Bandler. We felt on top of the world and empowered to make a difference with our amazing and guaranteed techniques. We guaranteed that if a client started smoking again, they could come back and see us free of charge until they stopped forever.

I was using the light and sound technology in my clinics. My father wasn't. Our advertising was bringing us on average 70 new clients a week in our clinics, which caused my father to hire three additional therapists to work with him. Me? I was handling the same number of clients on my own in my centers.

The only difference between how our clinics ran was that I was using the light and sound technology and recording my sessions with clients to take home for reinforcement. Once clients had my tapes to listen to at home, they had the opportunity to listen to the tones from the sessions as well as the brain-balancing music composed by Alexander McFee in the background. They were able to listen to the tapes all night long if they chose.

(You won't find any relics such as cassette tapes in our practice anymore, but you can use the next best thing--an mp3 player, the MindFit unit for brainwave entrainment, and streaming music from our www. self-masterytechnology.com site.)

Once my dad saw that the use of sound and light technology allowed him to get the same results much faster, he decided to expand the practice to include other things such as weight loss, phobias and stress control.

Needless to say, it wasn't long before we were able to set up every office with this technology and train every therapist we had to use it for personal and reinforcement sessions for our clients. In fact, at one time we had over 100 clinics across the United States and Canada using this technology to create change for thousands of clients.

The www.self-masterytechnology.com site has allowed us to launch our program to people around the world, helping to train medical doctors, chiropractors, hospitals, spas, NLP professionals and more to expand their practices with the latest brainwave entrainment technology.

How Light and Sound Supercharges Self-Help

Light and sound technology for brainwave entrainment helps us at a time when all else seems to fail. Our lives are spent trying to attain a balance between what is within us and what is in the outside world. Many people find it hard to balance the inner world with the outer one and some even resort to drastic measures to alleviate their discomfort.

Light and sound technology allows our minds to use substitute energy to expand our cognitive abilities for things like learning, insight, creativity, and especially to redirect our current psychological script. The reason the brain enjoys sessions like this is because it can undergo a large scale change via the relaxation techniques for which such technology is famous.

The effect of brain wave frequencies, as mentioned before, allow light and sound to be the perfect model for change to take place within the psyche. Since this technology operates on electric frequencies by cycles per second, or Hz, communication is possible with the brain as the light sends coded messages throughout it. Some brain cells are disposed to to this kind of energy. They can act as light transducers and can translate the flickering light stimulus for the brain.

Instant response is the result of such sessions, as the brain is required to function in different ways depending on the task at hand. If you want your creativity to improve, for instance, then this organ must activate the Theta wave levels and partner them with the Alpha brain

waves according to the desired outcome. If, on the other hand, rehabilitation is the desired outcome, then the brain waves must operate at
Delta levels to allow the growth hormones to be secreted.

Why is the MindFit the
Best Technology Today and for the Future?

Let's take a look back at what makes the consecutive use of light and
sound technology the breakthrough it is today. You see, even though
research has proven that both flickering lights and binaural beats have
the ability to produce a relaxed state of mind, it has also been discovered that light and sound technology combined can provide a more
consistent transition, almost 100 percent, through the brainwave
states--from Beta to Alpha to Theta and back to Beta.

The reason we mention this now is to explain an experiment we did
in the early days of this technology. We took 1000 patients from 30
different chiropractic offices and gave them the equipment to measure
the brainwave activity via a device called the Mind Mirror.

What we discovered was that a good number were actually able to
track their brainwave activity from the very first visit. These were the
meditators; people who were basically those that had previously practiced moving into altered states. The remaining participants were able
to accomplish this generally by the third visit.

By the time they entered this state, the brain had already moved
from a state of unconscious incompetence, as we discussed before, to
a state of conscious incompetence (meaning they now knew what they
didn't know before) and then into conscious competency (with the
ability to act on the new knowledge). From that point forward, they
were in a state of unconscious competency (where acting on the new
knowledge is easy and automatic). That means they allowed them-

selves to be guided or transported into a dreamy, drowsy state very near the threshold of sleep where they developed hypermnesia, or super memory.

Hypermnesia refers to a phenomenon where the amount of recalled information increases as the subject tries to remember something via a cyclic method. So it is through this method that they were able to imprint new things in their mind like thoughts and beliefs that can transform their lives, with future pacing to guide those changes into place permanently.

CHAPTER
THIRTEEN

The Wellness Revolution

Chapter Thirteen.

The Wellness Revolution

More and more people are seeing health as something that is whole body--not just physical. This Wellness Revolution is being led by the baby boomers, the first generation in history unwilling to accept aging and decline as their inevitable fate. Rather, they are proactively seeking out ways to maintain vibrant health and an active lifestyle well into older age.

Most physicians are unaware of this shift or that their role in society is changing from being a means to deal with disease and pain that is already there, to one of education to prevent pain and illness in the first place.

People are becoming more and more aware of their bodies and the fact that it's important to care for the body to prevent problems arising to begin with. They are looking to wellness practitioners because they are concerned with wellness, not sickness.

As an example, there are currently 35 million users of an online brain training program called Lumosity--with 100,000 new people signing up for the program each day. Lumosity is a neuroscience research company and they are experts in the field of enhancing cognitive brain performance through brain games.

The concept of Brain-Based Wellness continues to gain momentum thanks to the work of people such as Drs. Richard Barwell, Daniel Amen, Mark Hyman, Rob Melillo, Joe Dispenza, Rob DeMartino, Tim Merrick, Jared Leon, Francis Murphy, George Gonzalez, Ted Carrick and others. All of these people have been leading the charge to Brain-Based Wellness for some time and now is the moment to take control and learn to integrate it into our daily lives.

All of this comes back to the idea of Self-Mastery Technology or SMT. SMT stimulates the brain with the right combination of light and sound to release the right neuro-chemicals that help balance the brain. These are the chemicals that are naturally released when we have a pleasurable experience or when we're in a state of learning that causes our memory, concentration and creativity to improve.

Many of the algorithms that we're working with are those focusing on attention deficit disorders. The aim is to teach you to help your clients achieve full-spectrum brain wave activity, with Beta (for focus) still intact, so they will be able to interact with the world in a more relaxed mindset, getting the brain to work in harmony with the world.

To accomplish this feat, you could spend 20 years on a mountaintop with Buddhist monks learning how to meditate and focus your mind; but the reality is most of us aren't able to do that. In today's turned-on and tuned-in world, the only way to ensure the brain stays in full spectrum mode is to train it to do so using full-spectrum light and sound training. We need to ensure our brain waves are in balance. No one brain wave is superior to another. They all have essential function in our lives and balancing them is key.

SMT was originally developed to help people with chronic pain issues. It was found that when we are in pain our brains are stuck in Beta mode. In that state we're not balanced. The great thing about SMT is it helps the brain balance Beta, Alpha and Theta waves, thus allowing the body to create a pain-free state. It also helps create the proper flow of the neuro-chemicals through the brain and body; so that the body and mind are able to work together in harmony.

We've found that one of the side benefits of the brain and body being in balance is that innate intelligence is able to take over and wonderful, creative things happen. Incredible transformation begins to take place. The body naturally shifts into a healing state, enabling a more active lifestyle because the body is more relaxed.

What are the Uses of SMT?

By now you've realized how great this technology can be. The good news is that we've been able to hone our experiments since the time of the '80s and are pleased to announce that it has been highly successful with on of our primary targets--children. We discovered that once the brain is trained through accelerated learning, it can make the learning process much easier to handle.

Most people have the tendency of shutting themselves off to information if they think it will be too hard to learn it. We have a friend who teaches English to Spanish-speaking adults. She commented that her students' ability to learn English is directly linked to the attitude they hold upon entering the classroom. Those who cry and complain that it's too difficult or continually state, "English is too hard for me!" would end up living out that self-fulfilling prophecy. Those who entered the class with an eagerness to learn would invariably catch on quickly and advance rapidly.

We discovered that light and sound technology can actually change these kinds of negative thought patterns by allowing the subject to go into deep inner states of awareness that characterize change and lifestyle improvement.

We have helped people get rid of alcohol addiction through free programs. I was even sought out because of my connection with NLP (Neuro-Linguistic Programming) when I wrote my book, *"Awaken the Genius."* I also developed a program called *"Hidden Solutions,"* which was later transformed into *Awaken the Genius*, which focuses on teaching people to visualize and realize their dreams through the power of their mental faculties.

We have over 900 wellness health clinics around the world that are now using this technology. Many of our practitioners tell us that they not only use it for their patients but they also benefit from a session in the afternoon themselves, so when their evening patients come in to the clinic they are recharged and ready to do their best work--even though they've been there all day.

Statistically speaking, 20 minutes using Self-Mastery Technology is equivalent to three to four hours of good, sound sleep. It's equivalent to a session of meditation, although in reality you'd have to have years of training in disciplined meditation to have the same effect as 20 minutes of SMT.

Most people in meditation are not able to go deep into Alpha or Theta. They might achieve a few minutes at a time in this state, but for the average person that's about it. The problem is most people don't have the ability to focus at the level required to achieve this. Their minds wander and the minute your mind wanders, you are no longer in a meditative state and no longer achieving deep Theta or Alpha states. The amazing thing about SMT-style neuro-training is that we can track the brain patterns before, during and after use and see that the desired states are being achieved.

We sometimes refer to SMT technology as P90X for the brain. People tend to know how to create an exercise program for the body and understand its importance, but they are at a complete loss when it comes to exercising the most important part of the body--the brain.

For those of you unfamiliar with P90X, the program includes 12 intense workouts that use resistance, body weight training, cardio, plyometrics, abdominal work, martial arts, and yoga in conjunction with a nutrition plan, fitness guide and workout calendar. The developers of this program recognized that they could achieve superior results by combining the best of the different methods out there.

With SMT we took the same philosophy and applied it to brain wave entrainment. We combine neurosensory algorithms with psychoacoustics that trigger different parts of the brain and combine it with strategic mind-messaging--integrating language patterns, affirmations, and visualization exercises to stimulate positive, goal-oriented thinking. All of these individual pieces fit together to create a harmonic symphony for the brain.

We've tried to teach people meditation for 25 years and the most common complaint we hear is, "It's too hard. I can't sit still. I can't control my mind. I've got too many thoughts going round in my head at one time." These are all clues that you've got a brain wave imbalance and you need to bring your mind and body back into balance.

It's important to us that people are aware that this is not just a rising fad without any science backing our claims up. We've been doing this research on the brain for many years. In the last two decades alone we've seen vast improvements in computer technology and graphing programs that are able to track the brain waves of people experiencing SMT. With advancements in technology, we have been able to evolve from a unit the size of a microwave to a portable unit smaller than a deck of cards. This makes the technology a lot more accessible to a larger number of people. Technology continues to move and shift, and the end result is we will continue to improve our technology as advances allow us to do so.

Throughout the rest of this book we're going to show you how to utilize this technology yourself as you incorporate and implement it into your life. You will learn how to reach for your loftiest goals and more. By utilizing this system you'll gain a new sense of confidence and health. We believe it will truly benefit your life in ways you've never imagined.

FOURTEEN

The MindFit System
and SMT Audio Processes

Chapter Fourteen.
The MindFit System and SMT Audio Processes

Your brain is your most precious organ because it is your control center, meaning it controls every aspect of your life. Even when other vital organs keep working, without brain wave activity, the body is an empty vessel.

Modern science understands more about the brain than ever before. For instance, we now know that the brain is plastic—meaning that it can change itself, and does so based on the environment and input it receives. We now know that this is called neuroplasticity.

Neuroplasticity means that we are NOT victims of genetics or an imperfect IQ as once believed.

We all have the power of neuroplasticity. We can create our own successes by simply providing our brains the stimulus they need to transform us into mental powerhouses, capable of fashioning any life we desire.

You've heard us mention the MindFit system of brainwave entrainment throughout various chapters in this book and we've also talked a little bit about SMT; but now we're going to explain to you exactly what this program is and how it can work for you. This program is designed to help you overcome almost any problem and achieve just about any goal you set your mind to.

The innovators that created this program have developed 43 different audio series--and more are being developed at this time. Each one is specifically designed to imprint positive suggestions into the mind of the user and integrate them so they become positive habits.

These audio sessions are what you use to train your brain back into balance and help you achieve whatever goal you desire. Our favorite saying is, "You get what you rehearse in life, not necessarily what you intend."

We often tell people that conscious commitment leads to subconscious action. By learning this visualization process you will learn to rehearse the things that you want and desire. Remember, the subconscious cannot tell the difference between real and imagined, so by using the visualization process to imagine what you want, your problem-solving brain will find ways to make it so.

Once that is accomplished, you can begin to implement them into your life immediately, one day at a time. You will actually begin to think, act and respond as though the change has already been made, a natural part of your makeup.

Neuro-Sensory Algorithms (NSA)

The MindFit also uses a unique system that both enhances and modifies the mind to take on new possibilities of action and thinking patterns. These are called NSAs or Neuro-Sensory Algorithms. These are basically structured sounds that are able to modulate how the brain carries out complex tasks including emotional responses, shifts in attention, memory and especially sleep patterns.

The best thing about this system is that it can be used in almost any multimedia platform that employs sound as its medium. The MindFit is the perfect example of such a device since it uses light and sound technology in tandem to create the relaxation state.

There are machines sold today that can allow you to create your own light and sound pattern. However, my advice is to use one that has already been tested and proven and made by the hand of a professional. This is where the SILS, Sensory Input Learning System, which we told you about at the beginning of this book comes in. When this system was first developed it was up to the therapist to program the frequencies and guide the subject or client into the Alpha and Theta states of mind for relaxation.

Now, I was over the moon when Light and Sound Research successfully created the very first light and sound machine right in my own clinic in Scottsdale, Arizona. They started with a demo unit, but they weren't sure what its applications would be. That's when I asked them to let me use the device with my clients and see how it worked.

My clients all ended up loving the ten pre-programmed sessions. You can imagine the look on Larry and Linnea's faces (the owners of the company) when I asked if they could build ten more units so I could use them with more clients. Since that time they have repackaged and repositioned their technology to hone it to perfection.

This is similar to what we're doing with our Brainwave entrainment technology. By harnessing the power of mobile computing and the Internet, we're able to stream this breakthrough technology to all points around the world.

What are the MindFit's Clinical Uses?

We have constantly observed that a clinic's credibility instantly increases in the wellness profession once this technology is utilized in their clinical practice. That's because there is an increased interest in the medical field to claim the title of mind/body clinic. The truth is, clinics that don't integrate some form of measurable brainwave entrainment can be known as nothing more than body clinics.

Utilizing this technology in conjunction with the SMT audio series with the different wellness programs we offer benefits every person walking into that clinic. Today, Brain-Based Wellness is being utilized in chiropractic offices, wellness clinics and spas in increasing numbers—more than 1,000 worldwide at the time of this book's publication—allowing patients of these offices and clinics to make the most of whatever treatment they're receiving.

An Example: The Airline Industry Experiment

The alleviation of stress is the main focus of our experiments, which is why we felt the airline industry would be the perfect place to test our technology. Believe it or not, more than 25 percent of people are affected with aerophobia or a fear of flying. We believe the numbers could be higher since some people may not like admitting this fear. The whole experience of flying can be mentally and emotionally crippling to someone having to face this phobia on a regular basis.

How? This is where your body's internal clock or Circadian rhythm comes in. This refers to events occurring within a 24 hour period and is a basic system all organisms possess. As your environment changes, this clock entrains itself to the internal workings of the mind, which is especially observed in a light-dark cycle such as day to night.

If a person undergoes a constant environmental condition which is devoid of time cues, the rhythm of the clock usually displays a time period that is less or more than the normal 24 hours it should display. Since we have an internal clock that regulates our daily activities such as sleep and waking, we face difficulties readjusting it when we experience jet lag, sleep disruption, such as new parents often suffer, or untimely work shifts.

We discovered that light and sound technology such as our MindFit can help remove this phobia. This is why we developed the Sky Blue series to give airlines the perfect, soothing technology to settle the circadian rhythms in the body and eliminate the effects of jet lag. Several participants in our experiment also showed immense appreciation for the relaxation techniques that were characteristic of the strategic mind-messaging session.

Another Example? Cancer Clinics

We've also used this technology in cancer clinics. Nothing, absolutely nothing, is scarier than the fear, frustration and uncertainty that is part and parcel of a cancer diagnosis and the treatment of chemotherapy. Delta Oncology, in Norfolk, Virginia, utilizes our system to aid people that are undergoing this treatment to keep them in more positive states of mind. The Coping with Cancer series was designed because our clinical research shows that relaxation techniques help to boost the immune system while the patient works with his or her medical doctor.

In fact, we have an entire medical series that allows hospitals to use our audio sessions for both pre- and post-surgery. Remember, the brainwave entrainment was first designed as a means to reduce or eliminate the pain stimuli. We discovered that it could also be used to help ease the pain resulting from laser procedures and help eliminate the effects of varicose veins; a condition in which veins in the leg enlarge to painful proportions.

We have another program that helps lower blood pressure--but we have found regular use of the MindFit unit in general helps with this ailment as well.

What About Sports?

Good question and we have a terrific answer! What is more fun than watching a tennis match? Watching players who are motivated to win of course! We are pleased to report that the MindFit can also be used for sports enhancement, to give each player a mental coach that they can plug in and use whenever they feel the need for a little extra motivation.

Don't believe us? Take the golf legend, Tiger Woods, for example. Most people know that this pro has used hypnosis and employs a sports psychologist to helps him visualize successful shots. This helps him perform better on the green. Now, imagine a device that can actually synchronize and organize your mind in such a way that you can think, act and play like a pro yourself. That's what the MindFit can do for you.

Women's Health

Women have also benefited from our technology; especially when it comes to their health. We know how uncomfortable and painful--mentally and emotionally--menopause can be. Our Mind Over Menopause program helps women experiencing these life-altering symptoms to regain control over their own lives, as we teach them to master their brainwaves.

We have also successfully helped women go through Pain-Free Childbirth with this technology. There are a few who weren't able to be completely free of pain, but every one we've helped was able to reduce the stress during this critical period. This is the main reason why so many people are using the brainwave entrainment technology. Once stress is no longer an issue, they can get things done faster and more efficiently. How? By understanding that there is a connection between their mental state and their body's ability to manage the effects of this condition. These women are able to get a new lease on life.

Daily Aches and Pains No Longer an Issue

Remember what we said about doing a pain-free study at American Pain and Wellness? They are but one example of the many people who are using technology such as ours to overcome everyday aches and pains as well as age gracefully. As an example, a man in his mid-70s, who was president of his local rotary club, had decided to give up his position because he regularly had trouble forgetting words and his train of thought at the podium. His anxiety was palpable as he explained his fears about losing his mental capacity.

After just a few weeks of brainwave entrainment, he found that all of his problems at the podium had vanished. Had he been cured of dementia? Most likely, no. More likely, he had not been suffering from dementia at all. Rather, his fear of fumbling on stage had been putting him into such an intense state of fight-or-flight, all he could do once on stage was react to his fears, thus creating a self-fulfilling prophecy. Once his brain waves became balanced, the fear dissipated and he was able to speak from the platform with confidence and poise.

This kind of evidence speaks for itself. Using the MindFit has enabled people such as these to get more and better sleep, regain mental clarity, and strengthen their bodies against the ravages of daily stress that could make them fall apart otherwise.

Sales Mastery

A friend asked for a sales program using NLP some years ago. We agreed but only if he would utilize the brainwave entrainment with his workers as well, allowing them to take a wellness break during the day.

His sales people were responsible for going door-to-door to sell water purification systems that cost up to $5000. The key was to keep this price on the salesperson's mind so they could sell the system successfully to potential clients.

We developed a Sales Mastery Program to which each salesperson listened on a daily basis. We are proud to say that each employee that took part in our program demonstrated increased sales while they used the brainwave entrainment technology that we provided for them. The best thing was the owner didn't lose many employees during this time period since most of them reported enjoying their job more after utilizing and mastering brainwave entrainment.

People are now using this technology in sales settings around the world. Several professionals have learned to use their minds to improve the quality of their everyday lives by visualizing the sale in their minds first and then acting on it physically in the world. Through this technique, they are able to realize the success they've been looking for.

And More…

We have also used this technology in my clinics focusing primarily on weight loss, smoking cessation and stress reduction. I was recently commissioned to develop a series on Wealth Consciousness, by harnessing the buzz around *"The Secret"* and visualizing wealth in the mind first and then modeling your life pattern accordingly to get your desired result.

Just think! Even your friends, family and coworkers can benefit from the use of this science. Help them and help yourself by making use of this breakthrough technology.

Incorporating Brain-Based Wellness for Quicker and More Sustainable Outcomes

Natural, healthy and sustainable weight loss is a huge market in society today. In this section we're going to talk about how brain imbalance contributes to body imbalance and weight gain; and how to utilize Brain-Based Wellness to achieve health success.

Being overweight has surpassed smoking as the cause of the highest number of preventable deaths in the United States today. Two-thirds of adults are overweight, with one-third of those being obese. With so many weight loss programs out there, what's going wrong? Why are we not having a bigger impact on this epidemic? If we're looking at statistics over time, the percentage of overweight population in America continues to increase until it has reached epidemic proportions.

Why is this so important to realize? In most towns you can throw a rock and hit a weight loss center of one kind or another. The same is not true for a weight loss clinic that actually gets real, sustainable results in weight loss. In fact, we've found that whatever market we've been to, there has never been any real competition for our services, because there is no one out there addressing the mental and emotional sides of the equation and no one is able to get the results that we get because we do.

The average dieter ends up gaining weight instead of losing it over the long term. Most diets done cold turkey don't last over 72 hours. Many people start a diet on Monday to quit by Wednesday. Over the weekend they eat whatever they want, telling themselves they'll start a diet again on Monday. This habit turns into a vicious cycle. The average American woman by age 50 has spent 31 years of her life on a diet. That statistic is shocking and goes to show that traditional and commercial diet programs do not work.

As a country, we've focused on the health issues related to smoking and we have seen improvement as a result. The number of adults who smoke has dropped from 54% in the '80s down to 19% today. It's still not a perfect number, but it's vastly improved. As we said, obesity has now surpassed smoking as the number one preventable killer. With a growing epidemic on the horizon and no viable method for dealing with it, we offer a natural, safe and permanent solution.

Obesity leads to all sorts of healthcare conditions such as heart disease, diabetes and cancer. We also have to recognize that weight gain is a by-product of several issues, the first being that people are far more inactive than at any other point in history. With the invention of the computer and other technology we can do pretty much anything at the touch of a button from our couch. Our diets don't help this matter either. And we've already talked about how our overloaded and overstressed lifestyle contributes heavily to the blame.

There are hundreds if not thousands of weight loss programs out there, but none produce consistent results. Why? Because they're not getting to the root cause of the problem--the real reason people are overeating and not exercising. They try to change people's diets without changing their minds. On a typical diet, people will deprive themselves and restrict themselves of the foods they crave the most and within 72 hours they can't sustain it so they stop. They can't fight the ingrained brain wave patterns they've established through years of eating certain foods.

Most people want to exercise, know they should exercise, but they feel lousy and they don't have motivation to do it because, again, they haven't addressed the brain dysfunction that caused the problem in the first place. That's what we do. We teach you how to deal with it.

Stress has an immense impact on our weight and, as we discussed previously, stress is the most pervasive malady of our time, a "Silent Killer." We've also discussed how 90% of all illness is stress related according to the National Institutes of Health. The problem is that stress is not always felt as stress, but still goes straight to the body and attacks at the weakest points.

Finally, we need to recognize that pain may hurt, but stress can kill. That's an important factor to keep in mind. I know we keep saying it, but it's important to drive home the connection for those of you reading this book for the sake of your health. We're talking about taking things to the next level by getting the brain back in harmony with the body and the body to work with the brain. Once we achieve this, people can easily learn to think, act and eat like a naturally thin person, helping them to lose weight and maintain that weight loss for life. When the brain and body finally work in harmony, we can achieve great results.

Why Does Stress Have Such an Impact on Weight Loss?

Let's discuss how stress sets all this off. First, we have what's called the fight-or-flight response, which leads to what we've referred to and labeled as the Sympathetic Survival Syndrome. It has also been referred to as defense physiology because the body is constantly in defense mode. This system, as we are aware, is a genetic development of the body designed to help keep us from harm. It is innate intelligence at work. Remember, innate intelligence is all about our survival. Even though we're surviving through an innate process, genetic wisdom is working. The problem comes when we aren't given the opportunity to wind down and relax. We're trapped in the Sympathetic Survival Syndrome and that causes our body and mind serious problems.

This is another reason why diet programs have poor results overall. Diets, by their very nature, follow the principle that you make decisions on a conscious level. Most of us don't have enough time on a conscious level to think about better eating choices. We're in too big a hurry to spend any time thinking about what we're eating. So under that stress we revert naturally to our primitive behavior, the fight-or-flight response.

Everyone who starts a diet starts with the best intentions. You wake up in the morning with every intention to exercise and make healthy choices. But then stress kicks in--someone brings donuts to work--and before you know it, all the good intentions are out the window. This is why Brain-Based Wellness is so effective, because it's all about setting time aside to relax and be conscious and aware of what's going on in your environment and the world around you. It's important to do this to create the world you prefer first in your mind and then the body can settle and recover and start to believe it is possible. Then we can begin to live that truth out as we go through our day-to-day experiences. That's what Brain-Based Wellness is going to do for you easily and naturally.

We have clients who were lifelong members of Weight Watchers. The first question I ask them is, "Why would you want to watch your weight for the rest of your life?" Our philosophy is that it's better to simply think, act and respond like a naturally thin person--without having to think about it. Naturally thin people watch the food they consume naturally and without much thought, but they don't watch their weight. They don't usually even feel the need to weigh themselves. They have an image in their mind of their body and the body and mind work together to create the physiological effects necessary to achieve that.

When you're getting the right nutrition and the right psychological component, along with physical activity, true, permanent weight loss happens. This is how we get people to step off the diet roller coaster of losing and gaining. We teach them to take action and change their lives.

As we continue with the discussion of the fight-or-flight response and Sympathetic Survival Syndrome, we have to remember that too much fight-or-flight activity without corresponding rest and relaxation is what distress is all about. In today's highly stressful and fast paced world, it's not good enough to take a one minute break and expect your brain to suddenly become balanced. It doesn't work that way. So we constantly stay stuck in Beta mode and our brain is constantly racing. We've got to give our brains the opportunity to go into Alpha and Theta modes where it can relax the sympathetic nervous system and engage the parasympathetic system until we're back into homeostasis.

During fight-or-flight our adrenals go into overdrive. Most patients we see in our office have adrenal malfunction or adrenal exhaustion. This is why people are tired all the time. The chemicals they release to deal with stress--cortisol and adrenaline--set the body up for all kinds of serious problems. You can be feeling stress and feeling exhausted even if you are getting proper nutrition and supplements. Why? Because you need to balance the mind and the body chemistry. You need to give your body the best chance it has for innate intelligence, the super-conscious awareness that's a natural part of the body, to work with that nutrition so you can properly metabolize, digest and use it for energy.

Adrenaline

We have mentioned adrenaline previously. Adrenaline sends signals to the digestive system to decrease the activity of the stomach, primarily because digestion is not essential to immediate survival. Even though you may be taking all the right supplements and getting all the proper nutrition, if your body is in a constant state of fight-or-flight it won't be able to break those supplements down properly.

There's probably a good chance your adrenal glands are not working as efficiently and effectively as necessary as well. It could have to do with the types of foods you're consuming, but it also has to do with the levels of stress you're under. When you think about stress in relation to weight, you must understand that stress stimulates the hormones that regulate the body's desire for fats and carbohydrates. When our clients come to our practice and tell us that they're having a great day, having fun, doing the things they enjoy doing, they generally also tell me they're eating well. When things go bad and get stressful, generally the eating habits follow. Stress causes people to reach for the candy bar, the sweets, because they're looking for a sugar rush to make themselves feel better. They want to change their physiology by eating something unhealthy for their bodies and you only need to look around to see that that strategy isn't working.

Cortisol

When the cortisol levels and blood sugar levels in our body increase, insulin shoots up as well. For those of you unfamiliar with insulin, it is a fat storage hormone. Insulin tells the body to stop burning fat because its job is to burn up the sugar in the bloodstream. Cortisol, being the survival hormone that we discussed earlier, programs the body to store fat for future famines.

Fat in small amounts and of the proper types is beneficial. It protects you by helping to keep toxins out of your bloodstream. The downside of cortisol is that it will tell your body to store fat in the places you least want it--the belly, buttock, arms and thighs. This kind of adipose tissue can be difficult to get rid of once you create it. We've had patients that come to our clinic and tell us, "I'm running two to three miles a day and I'm still not losing any weight." This is because that running is stressing out an already overburdened body. To lose weight for life, you have to find the balance between healthy foods, exercise and relaxation. Unfortunately, there are dozens of exercise programs that overwork and stress out the body causing weight gain instead of weight loss.

Cortisol also increases the body's tendency to burn protein rather than fat. This is bad because your resting metabolic rate is now being altered. This means when the body is at rest it burns a certain number of calories each day. Protein burns the most calories when you're at rest. If you're taking away the protein from the equation, your metabolic rate goes down as well. This is what happens in most diet programs. People eat too few calories to sustain their activity level, which prompts a stress (cortisol) response. The body then stores fat and burns protein instead. It's like using kindling to keep your fire hot.

Cortisol is designed to signal the body to relax and refuel after periods of stress. Back in our primitive caveman days, cortisol's job was to keep us away from saber-toothed tigers and other dangers we could face. Today we have this same stress response all day long. Cortisol is released while we're on the road, at work, and at home watching CSI. We often have overweight patients who say, "I don't eat all day, but when I get home all I want to do is sit on the couch and eat." We call this the couch potato syndrome. All day long they are busier and busier and by the end of the day their bodies are screaming at them to rest and refuel. That's why they arrive home tired, lethargic and hungry.

We tell our clients that stress is more fattening than chocolate. We've all had people say they just have to look at chocolate to gain weight. Our theory is perhaps it is the stress of denying oneself the chocolate that is triggering weight gain. After all, of the top ten life stressors, dieting is ranked seventh.

How Are You Dealing With Stress?

I know we've been through the entire stress gauntlet and by now you have a pretty good handle on what stress can do to affect your life. Have you ever wondered what happens when you allow it to continually build up in your body? Once you let all that tension accumulate, you have the chance of building up a charge that can ultimately destroy you if you're not careful.

Think of a capacitor, for example. This device is meant to hold a charge, yes, but it has to discharge that stored energy via a circuit at some point in time, right? This is what happens to us as well. We all can hold onto stress for a certain limited period of time, but at some point we need to discharge that stress as well.

Why do you think that people who lead healthy lives have little, if any, stress related problems? They easily release that tension via regular exercise. Others, on the other hand choose to use debilitating methods to "release" stress such as alcohol, drugs and junk food. People like this tend to take their frustrations out on their families and friends when these methods ultimately fail to relieve their stress.

This is why the MindFit is just what the doctor ordered. Your wellness breaks are the perfect opportunity to let go of the worries of the day or take a break from that frustrating project you're working on. The MindFit allows you the time and energy to use the power of possibility and eliminate the stress from your life. Develop a life in which you come out on top and mold it according to where you want it to go using visualization and by realizing the benefits of a healthy life.

CHAPTER

FIFTEEN

What Can You Expect
by Practicing Brain-Based Wellness?

Chapter Fifteen.

What Can You Expect
by Practicing Brain-Based Wellness?

Did you know that we actually have three choices when faced with an uncomfortable situation? We can either face the situation head on or try to run away as fast as possible. There is a third solution, albeit an often overlooked one. We can choose to relax and interact with life using the unseen or other-than-conscious state of our minds to solve the problem.

Take a fighter pilot for example. This daredevil doesn't have a choice between flight-or-fight to begin with. They have to take control of their fears and relax enough to face the enemy within their sights. Some people do have the ability to dig deep inside their psyche and build resources and skills that can help them overcome fears and accomplish their goals.

By enhancing Alpha and Theta waves, you can experience the same focus they do and learn to tap into the infinite potential of your mind to uncover hidden talents. This cannot be achieved without balanced brainwave activity taking place. In the past, there was no way for anyone to get the brain out of high Beta levels if the person was under physical, mental or emotional stress.

The best thing about brainwave entrainment is that it doesn't care what you're thinking about. No need to raise your eyebrows. What we mean by that is this device has the ability to work with you and for you without you even being aware of it and regardless of what's going on around you or in your head. Everything is done passively. This can be likened to listening to classical music to make you feel relaxed. Conversely, you can listen to rock music if you want to feel motivated and fired up for a sporting event or to exercise. Either way, the music affects your brain without your conscious awareness of it.

As we mentioned before, brainwave entrainment technology exercises the brain into the intuitive or creative mind. It then delves even deeper into that part of the brain that is responsible for solving problems for you on a daily basis. Now, this is done with those skills that you think you never had, with resources you never knew existed. It's called potential, which is a crucial and hidden ability of the mind, which is responsible for helping us achieve our goals in life.

By using the other-than-conscious level of your mind to mentally experience the success you want to achieve, your mind will have an easier time placing the skills and resources you need on the timeline of your life. This will make those imaginary actions seem very real for you, making them extremely easy to implement into your life.

Let's take a trip through what an actual person goes through when he or she uses brainwave entrainment. The altered place that we just talked about is a very natural place for our minds to dwell in, since it shares similarities with what one experiences in the deepest sleep possible. It's actually very similar to what you experience when you're in the deepest states of sleep.

A Power Nap With a Purpose

The first thing that happens when you nod off is that your brain goes into a state that is between asleep and awake--or the hypnagogic state. It is then that the outer world seems to melt away, leaving you with a very strong awareness of the inner world of your mind. This is called Stage 1 sleep in which the mind is alert and conscious but the body appears to be asleep.

This is when brainwave entrainment allows you to move into the twilight state of awareness, where you're just about to fall asleep. You're basically dreaming while you're awake, which allows you to easily visualize and realize your goals. You become a child again, who has the unique ability to experience the creative part of his or her nature that most people refrain from indulging in when they enter adulthood. This is also when you start to learn how to solve problems by figuring out HOW to think rather than WHAT to think.

You move into a state of Theta after this occurs, where your body can activate its true healing state. This is where your mind goes when you're asleep since this is the part that rejuvenates the body as it slumbers. In other words, this is the state during which the body is reset according to the "blueprint" nature intended it to be--or the healthy state with which you started the day.

Brainwave entrainment will help you visualize these images even if you think you can't. How? The MindFit is fitted with special tone and light training frequencies that affect the frontal lobes of the brain in such a way that your mind creates a holographic experience for you. Your mind then uses that larger-than-life image to recreate pathways of your thinking processes and create new ones that can prove highly beneficial to you in the long run.

Utilizing untapped potential is the key to unfolding hidden talents and starting a whole new trend for your life. Brainwave entrainment will also ensure that those newly minted beliefs never leave the safe confines of your mind as it ingrains them into it every night as you doze off. It's very similar to a power nap, but even more effective because you are going there with a purpose.

In other words, you're being guided on the path to self-re-discovery. Instead of taking your old, outdated thoughts and beliefs to bed, you'll be able to think of and calculate new ones that have been created purely through the power of your own mind. All it really needs is a push in the right direction, after all.

We believe that anything worth doing well is worth doing poorly at first. The good news is you don't need to worry about doing anything poorly if you have brainwave entrainment working for you. Just as the fastest way to get from one state to another is by using a plane; the fastest way for you to reinvent your thinking processes is by retraining your brain.

Brainwave entrainment technology also gives one the intense relaxed state that is only possible if one has had thorough training with a Zen master. With as little as three sessions, you can reach that deep Theta state that is so necessary for actual healing to take place. However, what you do in that state is totally up to you.

What you can do is increase both your long and short-term memory as well as provide your attention span and concentration levels an upgrade. Each session also has the ideal healing effects that can reduce anxiety and eliminate depression, which are two debilitating states that stand in the way of every person on this planet.

The brain is the greatest pharmacy on earth capable of producing 30,000 different Neuro-chemicals as soon as a single thought runs through it. Imagine what you can accomplish once your mind is plugged in to access positive thoughts. You may even find it easy to reduce or eliminate medications, but be sure to do so only with the assistance of your prescribing physician.

Not only will that kind of mind power increase both the creative and logical sides of your brain, it can actually be made to visualize the results that you can integrate into your life. If you believe it, you CAN achieve it. Just think--like the geniuses of the past, even YOU can go to sleep with a problem and have a solution in your mind as soon as you wake up.

Since the mind and body are working together, you can even experience reduced levels of discomfort that you have previously felt on an everyday basis. Whether you suffer from headaches, muscle aches, nausea, or even PMS symptoms, if it's stress-related, brainwave entrainment can simply make them vanish from your psyche as if they never existed in the first place.

This newly restored balance in your life is very important if you want to spend your life satisfied with who you are and if you want the body to follow suit. Don't you want to feel the same? Practicing brainwave entrainment will make sure you do and will guide you on the path of discovery that YOU choose for yourself.

"Your body is designed to heal itself. The ability of the body to maintain its health and overcome illness is, in fact, among nature's most remarkable feats. But, you've been placed in a world that systematically interferes with this natural capacity, and your conscious involvement in your health is required if you are truly to prosper."
- Donna Eden and David Feinstein in Energy Medicine page 17

C H A P T E R
SIXTEEN

What Others Are Saying
About SMT and the MindFit

Chapter Sixteen
What Others Are Saying About SMT and the MindFit

Randy Clusiau's Story: "I'm 170 Lbs. Lighter!"

Thanks to Dr. Porter's Brain-Based Wellness program my weight dropped from an obese 350 pounds to an athletic 180 pounds. That's nine pants sizes. Most importantly, I've kept the weight off for six years--and counting!! I'd been overweight my entire life. I gained 100 pounds between the ages of 20 and 25 and just kept gaining. On airplanes I had to borrow the demo seatbelt just to buckle myself in. I had tried every crazy diet, fad, pill, gimmick and I'd read all the books and articles. I did the low carb diet and that seemed great at first, but as soon as I had one piece of bread I was done. I was 32 years old and if I didn't change my life I was going to have a heart attack before I turned 40. I needed to start by fixing the way I thought.

I started Dr. Porter's program as my New Year's resolution in the beginning of 2008. Instantly I slept better at night and my habits started changing. I drank more water without even thinking about it. After listening to one of my audio sessions I'd go to the fridge and automatically be drawn to the fruits and vegetables.

I lost weight like crazy that first year. Even when the weight loss slowed, I continued to see changes. I haven't felt this light since I was 17. I'm stoked! I had been eating to cope with stress, but now I've learned new ways to cope. I have a well-balanced lifestyle now.

The MindFit light and sound system is an amazing tool. I love listening to my sessions. It's my time to unplug from the world and to focus on myself, relax and lower my stress level. When you're super relaxed and focused, everything sinks in and you're able to solve your problems.

I've been able to reprogram my brain so the way I look at food and the way I look at life are different. That's why I'm confident I'm going to keep my weight off for good.

Doctors Are Getting Results

In 2006 we did a weight loss study with Dr. Scott Newman a chiropractor from California. When we asked him to put this technology into his clinic his first response was, "Well, where's your study?"

There have, in fact, been quite a few studies proving this technology, but we felt it would be helpful to do some of our own studies, especially in the area of weight loss. With Dr. Newman we did our own 12-week weight loss study. In our study we didn't provide any additional nutrition classes or supplements, but patients were provided regular chiropractic care. Patients listened to the sessions in what we call our Emotional Eating Series.

Over the course of 12 weeks, the average participant lost just over a pound a week without any other instruction. We provided no coaching sessions. We didn't tell them what to eat or not to eat. We just had them come in and listen to a session. That convinced Dr. Newman to implement Brain-Based Wellness into his own practice long term.

We conducted another study in Texas with a mixed medical group of doctors that included chiropractors as well as medical doctors. This group was called American Pain and Wellness, and with them we conducted a study on the brainwave entrainment's use with pain management. The study by American Pain and Wellness was comprised of 30 patients they had all had surgeries where some nerve damage had occurred that caused intense pain for which no amount of medication was helping.

The study was conducted over a 12-week period. During the study they found that over 80 percent of the patients were pain-free after the third week. However, they had the patients continue listening to the program to cement the changes in their brains and ensure the pain did not return. Half of the patients were able to remain pain free between each session. Ultimately, nearly all were able to manage their own pain at home, just by using the equipment, without the use of medication or any other intervention.

The current MindFit system we use is based on technology originally designed in the '80s for pain clinics. This technology works for pain because when you're in the relaxed states of Alpha and Theta, you feel no pain. Pain is only registered in the body when you're in Beta. If you greatly reduce Beta waves, the patient feels little or no pain or discomfort in the body. This is why certain people have what we refer to as a high pain threshold. Really what they have is a lot of Alpha and Theta waves and they are able to diminish or reduce Beta waves.

Side Effects

You may be wondering about side effects caused by this technology. The answer is there are no side effects. Utilizing this technology, you will sleep better, reduce stress and lose weight. There are no nasty side effects to deal with and especially not the kind associated with medications, such as sluggishness and addiction.

One positive side effect did occur during the pain study. It was found that on average the patients in that study lost just under a pound a week--with no weight loss suggestions within the processes they were listening to. That was great news and not a total surprise. You see, when cortisol levels are returned to normal, innate intelligence is able to bring the body back to homeostasis. The body goes to work dealing with the key issues that were ignored for so long. That means the program not only worked to reduce pain but it also helped them lose weight without even trying.

Do The Results Last?

It's all very well to talk about the results people get when they first start using SMT, but whether the results are sustainable is the real issue and probably the thing you're most interested in hearing about.

One of the things we've found with traditional weight loss programs is that people have the ability to lose weight. The challenge we encounter involves patients' emotional eating, stress eating, and habitual eating. Consequently, the majority of people can't maintain weight loss after they finish a traditional diet. This is something that is greatly improved when you utilize Brain-Based Wellness. Patients are now able to get great results and they are more successful at maintaining those results after the program ends. We're not talking about quick, fad results. We are talking about long-term, permanent results. That's what we need to aim for--results that get people thinking and acting like naturally thin people.

Dr. Patrick Keiran, a chiropractic physician from Jay, Maine had this to say:

I have been a happy PorterVision client since being introduced to the technology at a NeuroInfiniti training. When I first purchased MindFit, a primary goal was to enhance my intuition, clarity and effectiveness. I use it daily and know that my energy and clarity is now the same with the last patient of the day as it is with the first. Once my staff and I felt great changes, it was easy to engage patients as well. We've had dozens of patients use MindFit with our weight loss purification program. All have reported great changes in health, sleep, weight and energy, and many have stopped antidepressants and other meds. Because their habits changed by rewiring their brains with Self-Mastery Technology, most continued losing weight after the program was complete. Every chiropractor could enhance their results and expand the impact of their practice with this technology. Drs. Patrick and Cynthia Porter are the real deal and you will learn great neuroscience from them...please check out what they have to offer!

Richard Barwell, DC, the Founder of Neurologically Based Chiropractic and the developer of the Neuro-Infiniti biofeedback instrument says:

"In the world of neuroscience, staying up to date is critical in order to offer the best patient care. Dr. Patrick Porter continues to set new standards in neurological retraining. His latest product [MindFit] offers, once again, an advanced program in brain retraining and I am pleased to endorse his product. We have been able to test the brain response changes via the NeuroInfiniti EEG and demonstrate that it works as promoted. Nice work Dr. Porter!"

Q and A with an Expert - Dr. Jared Leon, DC

Jared Leon is a sensational chiropractor in Long Island, New York. He is a functional neurologist and he gets amazing results in his clinic. Jared also lives what we would refer to as the chiropractic lifestyle. He exercises regularly, eats healthy and nutritious food, takes supplements, gets adjusted regularly and he's one of the healthiest people you'll ever meet.

Q: You're using Brain-Based Wellness for yourself and your family and you're now incorporating it into your practice. Can you tell us why?

A: Initially, it started at a seminar. Dr. Porter was the guest speaker at a Lunch and Learn event and I was really excited about the potential of what he was saying and how it could be beneficial to my family, my practice and myself. I just decided to go ahead and give it a go at home. At the time, I was in the process of building a new office. I would use it almost every day--I'd say six out of seven days a week, sometimes twice a day. I was mostly using a lot of the creativity SMT sessions, as well as those for stress relief.

As I continued with the program, the most amazing thing started to happen. I was able to visualize in ways I could never have imagined before. I was seeing how to construct the new office, what the room layout would look like, how I wanted the colors and patterns, how it would all work together. I then brought the technology to my children, who were six and seven at the time. I had them use the Enlightened Children Series and the first thing my seven year old said to me was he felt so relaxed. We just continued to use it every day.

Once I had fully implemented the program in my family, I decided to create a Brain-Spa room in my practice. This was a room with a nice comfortable chair and a little table. I wanted to create space so it was almost as if you were sitting at home with the technology. The program is still attracting more and more patients to my practice and every day I'm letting more and more patients try it out.

Q: What kind of results have they experienced?

A: It's been really fun and exciting so far. I've had a lot of patients fall asleep really quickly. It shows how out of balance they really were. We just leave them and when the session is up we'll go in and wake them up. They're amazed by how they feel. Straight away they're asking when they can try it again.

Everyone has absolutely loved the technology so far and has felt substantially better and more relaxed. I ask them when they come back if they've been sleeping better after using the technology and every one of them has said yes. We've had great results so far.

Q: Have you encountered any resistance?

A: No. Nobody has given me any resistance. Nobody has said anything negative about the program itself. It's all been really positive.

It's Time To Change

Time is the most precious commodity that we have on this good Earth, which is why we want to personally thank you for the time you've spent with us reading this book. Each of us are given approximately 86,400 seconds to do with what we will each day. We would like to humbly thank you for utilizing those precious seconds, minutes and hours with us.

Why not log on to www.self-masterytechnology.com and discover our library of 577+ life improving titles to choose from. We guarantee you won't be disappointed. The final message we want to leave you with is we're here to help. Stay in touch with us at any time by contacting Dr. Patrick Porter at Patrick@portervision.com or Dr. Bob Hoffman at bob@themasterscircle.net. Feel free to ask questions, but take that first step towards utilizing Brain-Based Wellness to heal your life. This is an amazing journey and quite frankly, we've only just begun.

BONUS-CHAPTER

SEVENTEEN

21 Day Action Tracker.

Chapter Seventeen – Your 21-Day Action Tracker

Welcome to Your 21-Day Action Tracker. Let's get started with a brief explanation of how to use the tracking system. There are three unique days, and they repeat themselves for seven days each over the next 21 days. The idea here is to provide you a 21-day game plan to get your mind and body synchronized with the idea that you can eliminate stress, rid your body of frustration, and retrain your brain to work at optimum levels.

When you go through the Day One program, which will repeat itself on days four, seven, ten, 13, 16 and 19, you're going to start out by first evaluating your body and where you hold stress. Some people hold stress in the neck, some people in the abdomen and others in the jaw or shoulders. Do you immediately know where you hold your stress? If not, don't worry. With a little self-evaluation, you're sure to figure it out.

Once you identify where the stress is affecting you, you're going to evaluate it. Do you feel it as tension, aching or soreness, or has it evolved into pain? Are you able to easily release it? Does it release and come right back again?

By practicing methods of release throughout the 21-day protocol, you're going to start eliminating the stress sensations and feelings in that area of your body. When you look at the chart, you will see that your range is from one to eight. This is because we want you to be very specific, never middle of the road, so there is no middle choice. You have to pick either one, two, three, four, five, six, seven or eight. You'll notice there is no middle number. So you are on either one side of the spectrum or the other.

So let's take for example question one. How would you rate your current level of stress? The first day's answer will be your baseline. So wherever you are right now, in this moment, you'll circle that number. If your stress is intense and hasn't changed since reading the book then circle a one or two. If you've eliminated your stress already, congratulations. You're going to circle an eight. And as you go through this program, you will do the same thing for each of the different steps. No one else is going to see your answers or grade you, so you may as well be totally honest.

At the end of the chapter there is a key so that once you've filled in all the information you'll be able to graph your results. By seeing your results day in and day out--even though this is only a 21-day plan—you'll be developing a new sense of self-awareness and resiliency along with an inner calm. We're hoping you'll integrate this brain fitness model into your life for the rest of your life.

As you move through the series, you'll notice that each of the days has an audio-session associated with it. When you are following the day one structure, you're going to listen to "A.M. Number One." That's the focus session that you'll find on the PorterVision SMT app, which you can download for free from Apple's App Store or on Google's Play Store.

When you listen to that particular session, plan on it taking ten minutes in the morning. It's geared to increase your alpha and beta brainwaves so that you wake up your brain and you start to act in a recharged and revitalized way. Some people find that in the morning they feel a little groggy. This session is meant to shift the gears, clear the fog, get you into a productive mode, and get you out there taking action and accomplishing your goals.

You'll notice at the end of the day we'll recommend that you listen to the P.M. Program, which is, "P.M. Number One, Focus on Dreamtime," before bed. This session is designed to take you from the wide-awake states of Beta and Alpha and move you through Theta and drop you off into Delta so you have a deep, restful, relaxing, revitalizing sleep.

Now, if you already have the MindFit system, you're going to be listening to the sessions with it so you get the benefit of the light frequencies. Most people awaken at the end of the P.M. sessions just enough to remove the headset, turn it off, and place it on a nightstand. However, if you find that it's inconvenient for you to use the MindFit at bedtime, you can listen to the P.M. program with just earphones so you're able to fall off into sleep.

In the middle of the day, if you have the monthly app Streaming Service, we're going to ask you to select one session from one of the series. So if you're working on brain fitness, you're going to go to the brain fitness series. If you're working on stopping smoking, you'll go to the stop smoking series. If you're working on weight loss, you're going to do that with the weight loss series. Now, this is the same with each and every one of the three different sessions that you're going to be listening to.

So as you look over day one, you'll notice that each time you're going to be rating different activities and different sensations and feelings in your body. When you get to day two, you'll notice that the questions have changed. There is not as much rating. There is more dialogue going on. So every three days you're going to start to journal a little bit about what's happening to you. We're still going to have you listen to an A.M. program but this time, on day two, you're going to be listening to "A.M. Number Two--Concentration."

The reason we want you to rotate through the sessions, listening to number one on day one and then number two on day two and so forth, is we need that brain flexibility. We're trying to build those neural connections. So we've got to give you some variety along the way. Even when you're choosing your mid-day session, you will want to listen in rotation, starting with the first.

What we're asking you to do is quite simple, but it does take a little commitment on your part. Essentially, for 21 days we're asking you to listen to at least one hour of SMT sessions each and every day and then document those results.

We know that if you document the results day in and day out, what's going to happen is you're going to start to notice results that you never thought were possible, utilizing the internal resources you didn't know you had.

When you get to day three, you'll notice there is another grouping of different protocols that you're going to be evaluating from. For example, how have your body's old stress responses changed? You're going to note if it hasn't changed at all, has changed somewhat or you have eliminated all or some of it.

It's important that you document these things and be as honest and as open as possible so you can evaluate your changes and discoveries and what's happening from one session to the next.

Once you're done, what you're going to be able to do is look over the

21 days of discovery, where you're awakening your flourishing brain, and you'll begin to recognize just how unique you truly are and how you can utilize your thoughts to engage your brain and transform your life, not only for 21 days, but to integrate it into your life and the lives of your family and friends, because one thing is for sure, stress isn't going away.

But now you know there is plenty you can do about how it affects you, such as:

- Getting regular chiropractic adjustments

- Practicing deep breathing

- Getting no fewer than seven quality hours of sleep a night

- Eating a balanced diet and minimizing or eliminating sugar and caffeine

- Balancing your brain with Brain-Based Wellness Technology

- Staying fit and trim with regular exercise

- Maintaining healthy relationships

- Balancing work, rest and play

This 21-Day Plan is designed to be an adventure in self-discovery. It's a way for you to become more self-aware, not only of the stressors in your life, but also all that is positive and beneficial. The plan will help you evaluate how you improve within the first 21 day, with the hope that you will discover how easy living a Brain-Bases Wellness lifestyle can be, so you'll integrate it as a natural and normal part of your life experience, helping you de-stress, revitalize your brain and function at the highest level possible for you.

How exciting to know you can start living the life you prefer today, instead of the one you, perhaps, were dealt.

Best of luck on your 21-day journey and we look forward to hearing about your many successes!

Day 1 Date: ___ / ___ / ____
Chiropractic Adjustment Today? Yes or No

1) Where in your body do you hold or carry your stress? _____
_____
_____

2) How would you rate your current level of stress?

Hasn't Changed
1   2   3   4   5   6   7   8
                               (8) Eliminated

3) Time listened to AM01 Focus _____ . Please rate your energy after listening.

No effect
1   2   3   4   5   6   7   8
         (8) I am energized and ready for the day

4) Which SMT Session did you listen to: _____

5) How would you rate your relaxation during the session.

I didn't relax at all
1   2   3   4   5   6   7   8
         (8) I can't imagine going deeper

6) How "confident" do you feel about your ability to handle your daily stress?

Not confident at all
1   2   3   4   5   6   7   8
                           (8) Very confident

How "positive" is your attitude—in other words, how happy are you?

Very negative and unhappy
1   2   3   4   5   6   7   8
         (8) Very positive—couldn't be happier!

7) How much "energy" do you have?

No energy at all
1   2   3   4   5   6   7   8
                    (8) All the energy I want

8) How well do you "sleep"?

Not well at all
1   2   3   4   5   6   7   8
                    (8) Great—I'm well rested

9) How much "stress" do you feel in your daily life?

Very stressed all the time
1   *2*   *3*   *4*   *5*   *6*   *7*   *8*

(8) Stress-free: nothing bothers me

10) How would your rate your "overall health"?

Many serious health concerns
1   *2*   *3*   *4*   *5*   *6*   *7*   *8*
(8) My doctor says I'm in great shape!

11) How much "self-esteem" do you have and how many "compliments" do you receive?

No self-esteem at all/
No one compliments me
1   *2*   *3*   *4*   *5*   *6*   *7*   *8*
(8) Very high self-esteem. I get tons of compliments

12) Do you feel you get enough "exercise"?

No exercise at all
1   *2*   *3*   *4*   *5*   *6*   *7*   *8*
(8) Exercise daily

13) How would you rate the significant "relationships" in your life?

Very unhappy/
No relationships in my life
1   *2*   *3*   *4*   *5*   *6*   *7*   *8*
(8) Extremely happy/
My relationships are the highlight of my life

14) How confident are you that you will reach your ultimate goal?

Not confident at all
1   *2*   *3*   *4*   *5*   *6*   *7*   *8*
(8) Very confident

15) If less than 4 above, what stops you from being confident? _____

_____   _____

_____   _____

16) Observations from your day:

_____   _____

_____   _____

Listen to PM01- Focus In Dreamtime before bed.

Day 2 Date: ___ / ___ / ____
Chiropractic Adjustment Today? Yes or No

Please describe how your body's old stress responses have changed. _____
_____
_____

Please describe what your daily goals are as your stress level improves.
_____
_____
_____

Time listened to AM02 Concentration _____ . Please rate your energy after listening.

No effect
1   2   3   4   5   6   7   8
(8) I am energized and ready for the day

Which SMT Session did you listen to: _____

What action steps will you take after listening?
_____
_____
_____

What changed in your ability to handle your daily stress?
_____
_____
_____

Write any happy moments from the last 24 hours here?
_____
_____
_____

List any activies here that prove your "energy" is improving?
_____
_____
_____

List any victories over stress in your daily life?
_____
_____

Take a moment to list those things you are grateful for.

_____

_____

_____

List any compliments you received over the past 24 hours. Or, positive thoughts you have had about yourself or life.

_____

_____

_____

What type of exercise did you do today?

_____

_____

_____

What steps did you take today to improve the relationships in your life?

_____

_____

_____

Write one of your goals as if you have already accomplished it?

_____

_____

_____

_____

Observations from your day:

_____

_____

_____

Listen to PM02 Release Negativity.

Day 3 Date: ___ / ___ / ____
Chiropractic Adjustment Today? Yes or No

How has your body's old stress changed?
Hasn't Changed
1   2   3   4   5   6   7   8
(8) Eliminated

How would you rate your current level of stress.

Severe
1   2   3   4   5   6   7   8
(8) Nonexistent

Time listened to AM03 Motivation _____ . Please rate your energy after listening.

No effect
1   2   3   4   5   6   7   8
(8) I am energized and ready for the
day

Which SMT Session did you listen to: _____
How would you rate your relaxation during the session.

I didn't relax at all
1   2   3   4   5   6   7   8
(8) I can't image going deeper

How "confident" do you feel about your ability to handle your daily stress?

Not confident at all
1   2   3   4   5   6   7   8
(8) Very confident

How "positive" is your attitude—in other words, how happy are you?

Very negative and unhappy
1   2   3   4   5   6   7   8
(8) Very positive—couldn't be happier!

How much "energy" do you have today?

No energy at all
1   2   3   4   5   6   7   8
(8) All the energy I need

How well did you "sleep" last night?

Not well at all
1   2   3   4   5   6   7   8
(8) Great—I'm well rested

How much "stress" do you feel about your daily life?

Very stressed all the time

| 1 | 2 | 3 | 4 | 5 | 6 | 7 | 8 |

(8) Stress-free: nothing bothers me

How would your rate your "overall health" outlook?

Many serious health concerns

| 1 | 2 | 3 | 4 | 5 | 6 | 7 | 8 |

(8) My doctor says I'm in great shape!

How much "self-esteem" do you have and how many "compliments" do you receive?

No self-esteem at all/
No one compliments me

| 1 | 2 | 3 | 4 | 5 | 6 | 7 | 8 |

(8) Very high self-esteem. I get tons of compliments.

Do you feel you get enough "exercise"?

No exercise at all

| 1 | 2 | 3 | 4 | 5 | 6 | 7 | 8 |

(8) Exercise daily

How would you rate the significant "relationships" in your life?

Very unhappy/
No relationships in my life

| 1 | 2 | 3 | 4 | 5 | 6 | 7 | 8 |

(8) Extremely happy/
My relationships are the highlight of my life

How confident are you that you will reach your ultimate goal?

Not confident at all

| 1 | 2 | 3 | 4 | 5 | 6 | 7 | 8 |

(8) Very confident

If less than 4 above what stops you from being confident? _____

_____   _____

_____   _____

Observations from your day:

_____   _____

_____   _____

_____   _____

Listen to PM03 Creating Your Success Time-line

Day 4 Date: ___ / ___ / ____
Chiropractic Adjustment Today? Yes or No

1) Where in your body do you hold or carry your stress? _____

_____
_____

2) How would you rate your current level of stress?

Hasn't Changed
1   2   3   4   5   6   7   8
                                                          (8) Eliminated

3) Time listened to AM01 Focus _____ . Please rate your energy after listening.

No effect
1   2   3   4   5   6   7   8
                          (8) I am energized and ready for the day

4) Which SMT Session did you listen to: _____
5) How would you rate your relaxation during the session.

I didn't relax at all
1   2   3   4   5   6   7   8
                          (8) I can't imagine going deeper

6) How "confident" do you feel about your ability to handle your daily stress?

Not confident at all
1   2   3   4   5   6   7   8
                                          (8) Very confident

How "positive" is your attitude—in other words, how happy are you?

Very negative and unhappy
1   2   3   4   5   6   7   8
                          (8) Very positive—couldn't be happier!

7) How much "energy" do you have?

No energy at all
1   2   3   4   5   6   7   8
                                  (8) All the energy I want

8) How well do you "sleep"?

Not well at all
1   2   3   4   5   6   7   8
                                  (8) Great—I'm well rested

9) How much "stress" do you feel in your daily life?

Very stressed all the time
1   2   3   4   5   6   7   8

(8) Stress-free: nothing bothers me

10) How would your rate your "overall health"?

Many serious health concerns
1   2   3   4   5   6   7   8
(8) My doctor says I'm in great shape!

11) How much "self-esteem" do you have and how many "compliments" do you receive?

No self-esteem at all/
No one compliments me
1   2   3   4   5   6   7   8
(8) Very high self-esteem. I get tons of compliments

12) Do you feel you get enough "exercise"?

No exercise at all
1   2   3   4   5   6   7   8
(8) Exercise daily

13) How would you rate the significant "relationships" in your life?

Very unhappy/
No relationships in my life
1   2   3   4   5   6   7   8
(8) Extremely happy/
My relationships are the highlight of my life

14) How confident are you that you will reach your ultimate goal?

Not confident at all
1   2   3   4   5   6   7   8
(8) Very confident

15) If less than 4 above, what stops you from being confident? _____
_____ _____
_____ _____

16) Observations from your day:
_____ _____
_____ _____
_____ _____

Listen to PM01- Focus In Dreamtime before bed.

Day 5 Date: ___ / ___ / ____
Chiropractic Adjustment Today? Yes or No

Please describe how your body's old stress responses have changed. _____

_____

_____

Please describe what your daily goals are as your stress level improves.

_____

_____

_____

Time listened to AM02 Concentration _____ . *Please rate your energy after listening.*

No effect

1 2 3 4 5 6 7 8

(8) I am energized and ready for the day

Which SMT Session did you listen to: _____

What action steps will you take after listening?

_____

_____

_____

What changed in your ability to handle your daily stress?

_____

_____

_____

Write any happy moments from the last 24 hours here?

_____

_____

_____

List any activies here that prove your "energy" is improving?

_____

_____

_____

List any victories over stress in your daily life?

_____

_____

Take a moment to list those things you are grateful for.

_____

_____

_____

List any compliments you received over the past 24 hours. Or, positive thoughts you have had about yourself or life.

_____

_____

_____

What type of exercise did you do today?

_____

_____

_____

What steps did you take today to improve the relationships in your life?

_____

_____

_____

Write one of your goals as if you have already accomplished it?

_____

_____

_____

_____

Observations from your day:

_____

_____

_____

_____

Listen to PM02 Release Negativity.

Day 6 Date: ___ / ___ / ____
Chiropractic Adjustment Today? Yes or No

How has your body's old stress changed?
Hasn't Changed
| 1 | 2 | 3 | 4 | 5 | 6 | 7 | 8 |
(8) Eliminated

How would you rate your current level of stress.

Severe
| 1 | 2 | 3 | 4 | 5 | 6 | 7 | 8 |
(8) Nonexistent

Time listened to AM03 Motivation _____ . Please rate your energy after listening.

No effect
| 1 | 2 | 3 | 4 | 5 | 6 | 7 | 8 |
(8) I am energized and ready for the day

Which SMT Session did you listen to: _____
How would you rate your relaxation during the session.

I didn't relax at all
| 1 | 2 | 3 | 4 | 5 | 6 | 7 | 8 |
(8) I can't image going deeper

How "confident" do you feel about your ability to handle your daily stress?

Not confident at all
| 1 | 2 | 3 | 4 | 5 | 6 | 7 | 8 |
(8) Very confident

How "positive" is your attitude—in other words, how happy are you?

Very negative and unhappy
| 1 | 2 | 3 | 4 | 5 | 6 | 7 | 8 |
(8) Very positive—couldn't be happier!

How much "energy" do you have today?

No energy at all
| 1 | 2 | 3 | 4 | 5 | 6 | 7 | 8 |
(8) All the energy I need

How well did you "sleep" last night?

Not well at all
| 1 | 2 | 3 | 4 | 5 | 6 | 7 | 8 |
(8) Great—I'm well rested

How much "stress" do you feel about your daily life?

Very stressed all the time
1   2   3   4   5   6   7   8
                                    (8) Stress-free: nothing bothers me

How would your rate your "overall health" outlook?

Many serious health concerns
1   2   3   4   5   6   7   8
                                    (8) My doctor says I'm in great shape!

How much "self-esteem" do you have and how many "compliments" do you receive?

No self-esteem at all/
No one compliments me
1   2   3   4   5   6   7   8
                        (8) Very high self-esteem. I get tons of compliments.

Do you feel you get enough "exercise"?

No exercise at all
1   2   3   4   5   6   7   8
                                                    (8) Exercise daily

How would you rate the significant "relationships" in your life?

Very unhappy/
No relationships in my life
1   2   3   4   5   6   7   8
                                    (8) Extremely happy/
                        My relationships are the highlight of my life

How confident are you that you will reach your ultimate goal?

Not confident at all
1   2   3   4   5   6   7   8
                                            (8) Very confident

If less than 4 above what stops you from being confident? _____

_____ _____
_____ _____

Observations from your day:

_____ _____
_____ _____

Listen to PM03 Creating Your Success Time-line

Day 7 Date: ___ / ___ / ____
Chiropractic Adjustment Today? Yes or No

1) Where in your body do you hold or carry your stress? _____

_____

2) How would you rate your current level of stress?

Hasn't Changed
1   2   3   4   5   6   7   8
                                                                Eliminated

3) Time listened to AM01 Focus _____ . *Please rate your energy after listening.*

No effect
1   2   3   4   5   6   7   8
                                    (8) I am energized and ready for the day

4) Which SMT Session did you listen to: _____
5) How would you rate your relaxation during the session.

I didn't relax at all
1   2   3   4   5   6   7   8
                                        (8) I can't imagine going deeper

6) How "confident" do you feel about your ability to handle your daily stress?

Not confident at all
1   2   3   4   5   6   7   8
                                                    (8) Very confident

How "positive" is your attitude—in other words, how happy are you?

Very negative and unhappy
1   2   3   4   5   6   7   8
                                (8) Very positive—couldn't be happier!

7) How much "energy" do you have?

No energy at all
1   2   3   4   5   6   7   8
                                                (8) All the energy I want

8) How well do you "sleep"?

Not well at all
1   2   3   4   5   6   7   8
                                            (8) Great—I'm well rested

9) How much "stress" do you feel in your daily life?

Very stressed all the time
1   2   3   4   5   6   7   8

(8) Stress-free: nothing bothers me

10) How would your rate your "overall health"?

Many serious health concerns
1   2   3   4   5   6   7   8
(8) My doctor says I'm in great shape!

11) How much "self-esteem" do you have and how many "compliments" do you receive?

No self-esteem at all/
No one compliments me
1   2   3   4   5   6   7   8
(8) Very high self-esteem. I get tons of compliments

12) Do you feel you get enough "exercise"?

No exercise at all
1   2   3   4   5   6   7   8
(8) Exercise daily

13) How would you rate the significant "relationships" in your life?

Very unhappy/
No relationships in my life
1   2   3   4   5   6   7   8
(8) Extremely happy/
My relationships are the highlight of my life

14) How confident are you that you will reach your ultimate goal?

Not confident at all
1   2   3   4   5   6   7   8
(8) Very confident

15) If less than 4 above, what stops you from being confident? _____

_____ _____

_____ _____

16) Observations from your day:

_____ _____

_____ _____

_____ _____

Listen to PM01- Focus In Dreamtime before bed.

Day 8 Date: ___ / ___ / ____
Chiropractic Adjustment Today? Yes or No

Please describe how your body's old stress responses have changed. _____

_____

_____

Please describe what your daily goals are as your stress level improves.

_____

_____

_____

Time listened to AM02 Concentration _____ . Please rate your energy after listening.

No effect
1   2   3   4   5   6   7   8
                              (8) I am energized and ready for the day

Which SMT Session did you listen to: _____

What action steps will you take after listening?

_____

_____

_____

What changed in your ability to handle your daily stress?

_____

_____

_____

Write any happy moments from the last 24 hours here?

_____

_____

_____

List any activies here that prove your "energy" is improving?

_____

_____

_____

List any victories over stress in your daily life?

_____

_____

Take a moment to list those things you are grateful for.

_____
_____
_____

List any compliments you received over the past 24 hours. Or, positive thoughts you have had about yourself or life.

_____
_____
_____

What type of exercise did you do today?

_____
_____
_____

What steps did you take today to improve the relationships in your life?

_____
_____
_____

Write one of your goals as if you have already accomplished it?

_____
_____
_____
_____

Observations from your day:

_____
_____
_____
_____

Listen to PM02 Release Negativity.

Day 9 Date: ___ / ___ / ____
Chiropractic Adjustment Today? Yes or No

How has your body's old stress changed?
Hasn't Changed
| 1 | 2 | 3 | 4 | 5 | 6 | 7 | 8 |

(8) Eliminated

How would you rate your current level of stress.

Severe
| 1 | 2 | 3 | 4 | 5 | 6 | 7 | 8 |

(8) Nonexistent

Time listened to AM03 Motivation _____ . Please rate your energy after listening.

No effect
| 1 | 2 | 3 | 4 | 5 | 6 | 7 | 8 |

(8) I am energized and ready for the day

Which SMT Session did you listen to: _____
How would you rate your relaxation during the session.

I didn't relax at all
| 1 | 2 | 3 | 4 | 5 | 6 | 7 | 8 |

(8) I can't image going deeper

How "confident" do you feel about your ability to handle your daily stress?

Not confident at all
| 1 | 2 | 3 | 4 | 5 | 6 | 7 | 8 |

(8) Very confident

How "positive" is your attitude—in other words, how happy are you?

Very negative and unhappy
| 1 | 2 | 3 | 4 | 5 | 6 | 7 | 8 |

(8) Very positive—couldn't be happier!

How much "energy" do you have today?

No energy at all
| 1 | 2 | 3 | 4 | 5 | 6 | 7 | 8 |

(8) All the energy I need

How well did you "sleep" last night?

Not well at all
| 1 | 2 | 3 | 4 | 5 | 6 | 7 | 8 |

(8) Great—I'm well rested

How much "stress" do you feel about your daily life?

Very stressed all the time
1   2   3   4   5   6   7   8

(8) Stress-free: nothing bothers me

How would your rate your "overall health" outlook?

Many serious health concerns
1   2   3   4   5   6   7   8

(8) My doctor says I'm in great shape!

How much "self-esteem" do you have and how many "compliments" do you receive?

No self-esteem at all/
No one compliments me
1   2   3   4   5   6   7   8

(8) Very high self-esteem. I get tons of compliments.

Do you feel you get enough "exercise"?

No exercise at all
1   2   3   4   5   6   7   8

(8) Exercise daily

How would you rate the significant "relationships" in your life?

Very unhappy/
No relationships in my life
1   2   3   4   5   6   7   8

(8) Extremely happy/
My relationships are the highlight of my life

How confident are you that you will reach your ultimate goal?

Not confident at all
1   2   3   4   5   6   7   8

(8) Very confident

If less than 4 above what stops you from being confident? _____

_____ _____

_____ _____

Observations from your day:

_____ _____

_____ _____

_____ _____

Listen to PM03 Creating Your Success Time-line

Day 10 Date: ___ / ___ / _____
Chiropractic Adjustment Today? Yes or No

1) Where in your body do you hold or carry your stress? _____

_____

_____

2) How would you rate your current level of stress?

Hasn't Changed
1   2   3   4   5   6   7   8
                                    Eliminated

3) Time listened to AM01 Focus _____ . *Please rate your energy after listening.*

No effect
1   2   3   4   5   6   7   8
                            (8) I am energized and ready for the day

4) Which SMT Session did you listen to: _____
5) How would you rate your relaxation during the session.

I didn't relax at all
1   2   3   4   5   6   7   8
                        (8) I can't imagine going deeper

6) How "confident" do you feel about your ability to handle your daily stress?

Not confident at all
1   2   3   4   5   6   7   8
                            (8) Very confident

How "positive" is your attitude—in other words, how happy are you?

Very negative and unhappy
1   2   3   4   5   6   7   8
                      (8) Very positive—couldn't be happier!

7) How much "energy" do you have?

No energy at all
1   2   3   4   5   6   7   8
                          (8) All the energy I want

8) How well do you "sleep"?

Not well at all
1   2   3   4   5   6   7   8
                        (8) Great—I'm well rested

9) How much "stress" do you feel in your daily life?

Very stressed all the time
1   2   3   4   5   6   7   8
(8) Stress-free: nothing bothers me

10) How would your rate your "overall health"?

Many serious health concerns
1   2   3   4   5   6   7   8
(8) My doctor says I'm in great shape!

11) How much "self-esteem" do you have and how many "compliments" do you receive?

No self-esteem at all/
No one compliments me
1   2   3   4   5   6   7   8
(8) Very high self-esteem. I get tons of compliments

12) Do you feel you get enough "exercise"?

No exercise at all
1   2   3   4   5   6   7   8
(8) Exercise daily

13) How would you rate the significant "relationships" in your life?

Very unhappy/
No relationships in my life
1   2   3   4   5   6   7   8
(8) Extremely happy/
My relationships are the highlight of my life

14) How confident are you that you will reach your ultimate goal?

Not confident at all
1   2   3   4   5   6   7   8
(8) Very confident

15) If less than 4 above, what stops you from being confident? _____

_____ _____

_____ _____

16) Observations from your day:

_____ _____

_____ _____

_____ _____

Listen to PM01- Focus In Dreamtime before bed.

Day 11 Date: ___ / ___ / ____
Chiropractic Adjustment Today? Yes or No

Please describe how your body's old stress responses have changed. _____
_____
_____

Please describe what your daily goals are as your stress level improves.
_____
_____
_____

Time listened to AM02 Concentration _____ *. Please rate your energy after listening.*

No effect
1   2   3   4   5   6   7   8
(8) I am energized and ready for the day

Which SMT Session did you listen to: _____

What action steps will you take after listening?
_____
_____
_____

What changed in your ability to handle your daily stress?
_____
_____
_____

Write any happy moments from the last 24 hours here?
_____
_____
_____

List any activies here that prove your "energy" is improving?
_____
_____
_____

List any victories over stress in your daily life?
_____
_____

Take a moment to list those things you are grateful for.

_____
_____
_____

List any compliments you received over the past 24 hours. Or, positive thoughts you have had about yourself or life.

_____
_____
_____

What type of exercise did you do today?

_____
_____
_____

What steps did you take today to improve the relationships in your life?

_____
_____
_____

Write one of your goals as if you have already accomplished it?

_____
_____
_____
_____

Observations from your day:

_____
_____
_____
_____

Listen to PM02 Release Negativity.

Day 12 Date: ___ / ___ / ____
Chiropractic Adjustment Today? Yes or No

How has your body's old stress changed?
Hasn't Changed
1   2   3   4   5   6   7   8
(8) Eliminated

How would you rate your current level of stress.

Severe
1   2   3   4   5   6   7   8
(8) Nonexistent

Time listened to AM03 Motivation _____ . *Please rate your energy after listening.*

No effect
1   2   3   4   5   6   7   8
(8) I am energized and ready for the day

Which SMT Session did you listen to: _____
How would you rate your relaxation during the session.

I didn't relax at all
1   2   3   4   5   6   7   8
(8) I can't image going deeper

How "confident" do you feel about your ability to handle your daily stress?

Not confident at all
1   2   3   4   5   6   7   8
(8) Very confident

How "positive" is your attitude—in other words, how happy are you?

Very negative and unhappy
1   2   3   4   5   6   7   8
(8) Very positive—couldn't be happier!

How much "energy" do you have today?

No energy at all
1   2   3   4   5   6   7   8
(8) All the energy I need

How well did you "sleep" last night?

Not well at all
1   2   3   4   5   6   7   8
(8) Great—I'm well rested

How much "stress" do you feel about your daily life?

Very stressed all the time
1   2   3   4   5   6   7   8

(8) Stress-free: nothing bothers me

How would your rate your "overall health" outlook?

Many serious health concerns
1   2   3   4   5   6   7   8

(8) My doctor says I'm in great shape!

How much "self-esteem" do you have and how many "compliments" do you receive?

No self-esteem at all/
No one compliments me
1   2   3   4   5   6   7   8

(8) Very high self-esteem. I get tons of compliments

Do you feel you get enough "exercise"?

No exercise at all
1   2   3   4   5   6   7   8

(8) Exercise daily

How would you rate the significant "relationships" in your life?

Very unhappy/
No relationships in my life
1   2   3   4   5   6   7   8

(8) Extremely happy/
My relationships are the highlight of my life

How confident are you that you will reach your ultimate goal?

Not confident at all
1   2   3   4   5   6   7   8

(8) Very confident

If less than 4 above what stops you from being confident? _____
_____   _____
_____   _____

Observations from your day:
_____   _____
_____   _____
_____   _____

Listen to PM03 Creating Your Success Time-line

Day 13 Date: ___ / ___ / ____
Chiropractic Adjustment Today? Yes or No

1) Where in your body do you hold or carry your stress? _____
_____
_____

2) How would you rate your current level of stress?

Hasn't Changed
1   2   3   4   5   6   7   8
                                              (8) Eliminated

3) Time listened to AM01 Focus _____ . Please rate your energy after listening.

No effect
1   2   3   4   5   6   7   8
                        (8) I am energized and ready for the day

4) Which SMT Session did you listen to: _____
5) How would you rate your relaxation during the session.

I didn't relax at all
1   2   3   4   5   6   7   8
                              (8) I can't imagine going deeper

6) How "confident" do you feel about your ability to handle your daily stress?

Not confident at all
1   2   3   4   5   6   7   8
                                         (8) Very confident

How "positive" is your attitude—in other words, how happy are you?

Very negative and unhappy
1   2   3   4   5   6   7   8
                        (8) Very positive—couldn't be happier!

7) How much "energy" do you have?

No energy at all
1   2   3   4   5   6   7   8
                                    (8) All the energy I want

8) How well do you "sleep"?

Not well at all
1   2   3   4   5   6   7   8
                                  (8) Great—I'm well rested

9) How much "stress" do you feel in your daily life?

Very stressed all the time
1   *2*   *3*   *4*   *5*   *6*   *7*   *8*

(8) Stress-free: nothing bothers me

10) How would your rate your "overall health"?

Many serious health concerns
1   *2*   *3*   *4*   *5*   *6*   *7*   *8*
(8) My doctor says I'm in great shape!

11) How much "self-esteem" do you have and how many "compliments" do you receive?

No self-esteem at all/
No one compliments me
1   *2*   *3*   *4*   *5*   *6*   *7*   *8*
(8) Very high self-esteem. I get tons of compliments

12) Do you feel you get enough "exercise"?

No exercise at all
1   *2*   *3*   *4*   *5*   *6*   *7*   *8*
(8) Exercise daily

13) How would you rate the significant "relationships" in your life?

Very unhappy/
No relationships in my life
1   *2*   *3*   *4*   *5*   *6*   *7*   *8*
(8) Extremely happy/
My relationships are the highlight of my life

14) How confident are you that you will reach your ultimate goal?

Not confident at all
1   *2*   *3*   *4*   *5*   *6*   *7*   *8*
(8) Very confident

15) If less than 4 above, what stops you from being confident? _____

_____ _____
_____ _____

16) Observations from your day:

_____ _____
_____ _____
_____ _____

Listen to PM01- Focus In Dreamtime before bed.

Day 14 Date: ___ / ___ / ____
Chiropractic Adjustment Today? Yes or No

Please describe how your body's old stress responses have changed. _____

_____

_____

Please describe what your daily goals are as your stress level improves.

_____

_____

_____

Time listened to AM02 Concentration _____ . Please rate your energy after listening.

No effect
1   2   3   4   5   6   7   8
                                        (8) I am energized and ready for the day

Which SMT Session did you listen to: _____

What action steps will you take after listening?

_____

_____

_____

What changed in your ability to handle your daily stress?

_____

_____

_____

Write any happy moments from the last 24 hours here?

_____

_____

_____

List any activies here that prove your "energy" is improving?

_____

_____

_____

List any victories over stress in your daily life?

_____

_____

Take a moment to list those things you are grateful for.

_____

_____

_____

List any compliments you received over the past 24 hours. Or, positive thoughts you have had about yourself or life.

_____

_____

_____

What type of exercise did you do today?

_____

_____

_____

What steps did you take today to improve the relationships in your life?

_____

_____

_____

Write one of your goals as if you have already accomplished it?

_____

_____

_____

_____

Observations from your day:

_____

_____

_____

_____

Listen to PM02 Release Negativity.

Day 15 Date: ___ / ___ / ____
Chiropractic Adjustment Today? Yes or No

How has your body's old stress changed?
Hasn't Changed
1   2   3   4   5   6   7   8
(8) Eliminated

How would you rate your current level of stress.
Severe
1   2   3   4   5   6   7   8
(8) Nonexistent

Time listened to AM03 Motivation _____ . Please rate your energy after listening.
No effect
1   2   3   4   5   6   7   8
(8) I am energized and ready for the day

Which SMT Session did you listen to: _____
How would you rate your relaxation during the session.
I didn't relax at all
1   2   3   4   5   6   7   8
(8) I can't image going deeper

How "confident" do you feel about your ability to handle your daily stress?
Not confident at all
1   2   3   4   5   6   7   8
(8) Very confident

How "positive" is your attitude—in other words, how happy are you?
Very negative and unhappy
1   2   3   4   5   6   7   8
(8) Very positive—couldn't be happier!

How much "energy" do you have today?
No energy at all
1   2   3   4   5   6   7   8
(8) All the energy I need

How well did you "sleep" last night?
Not well at all
1   2   3   4   5   6   7   8
(8) Great—I'm well rested

How much "stress" do you feel about your daily life?

Very stressed all the time
1   2   3   4   5   6   7   8

(8) Stress-free: nothing bothers me

How would your rate your "overall health" outlook?

Many serious health concerns
1   2   3   4   5   6   7   8

(8) My doctor says I'm in great shape!

How much "self-esteem" do you have and how many "compliments" do you receive?

No self-esteem at all/
No one compliments me
1   2   3   4   5   6   7   8

(8) Very high self-esteem. I get tons of compliments

Do you feel you get enough "exercise"?

No exercise at all
1   2   3   4   5   6   7   8

(8) Exercise daily

How would you rate the significant "relationships" in your life?

Very unhappy/
No relationships in my life
1   2   3   4   5   6   7   8

(8) Extremely happy/
My relationships are the highlight of my life

How confident are you that you will reach your ultimate goal?

Not confident at all
1   2   3   4   5   6   7   8

(8) Very confident

If less than 4 above what stops you from being confident? _____

_____ _____
_____ _____

Observations from your day:

_____ _____
_____ _____
_____ _____

Listen to PM03 Creating Your Success Time-line

Day 16 Date: ___ / ___ / ____
Chiropractic Adjustment Today? Yes or No

1) Where in your body do you hold or carry your stress? _____

_____

2) How would you rate your current level of stress?

Hasn't Changed
1   2   3   4   5   6   7   8
                                                      (8) Eliminated

3) Time listened to AM01 Focus _____ . Please rate your energy after listening.

No effect
1   2   3   4   5   6   7   8
                              (8) I am energized and ready for the day

4) Which SMT Session did you listen to: _____

5) How would you rate your relaxation during the session.

I didn't relax at all
1   2   3   4   5   6   7   8
                              (8) I can't imagine going deeper

6) How "confident" do you feel about your ability to handle your daily stress?

Not confident at all
1   2   3   4   5   6   7   8
                                              (8) Very confident

How "positive" is your attitude—in other words, how happy are you?

Very negative and unhappy
1   2   3   4   5   6   7   8
                              (8) Very positive—couldn't be happier!

7) How much "energy" do you have?

No energy at all
1   2   3   4   5   6   7   8
                                      (8) All the energy I want

8) How well do you "sleep"?

Not well at all
1   2   3   4   5   6   7   8
                                      (8) Great—I'm well rested

9) How much "stress" do you feel in your daily life?

Very stressed all the time
1   2   3   4   5   6   7   8

                                                (8) Stress-free: nothing bothers me

10) How would your rate your "overall health"?

Many serious health concerns
1   2   3   4   5   6   7   8
                                        (8) My doctor says I'm in great shape!

11) How much "self-esteem" do you have and how many "compliments" do you receive?

No self-esteem at all/
No one compliments me
1   2   3   4   5   6   7   8
                                (8) Very high self-esteem. I get tons of compliments

12) Do you feel you get enough "exercise"?

No exercise at all
1   2   3   4   5   6   7   8
                                                        (8) Exercise daily

13) How would you rate the significant "relationships" in your life?

Very unhappy/
No relationships in my life
1   2   3   4   5   6   7   8
                                                        (8) Extremely happy/
                                        My relationships are the highlight of my life

14) How confident are you that you will reach your ultimate goal?

Not confident at all
1   2   3   4   5   6   7   8
                                                        (8) Very confident

15) If less than 4 above, what stops you from being confident? _____

_____   _____

_____   _____

16) Observations from your day:

_____   _____

_____   _____

_____   _____

Listen to PM01- Focus In Dreamtime before bed.

Day 17 Date: ___ / ___ / ____
Chiropractic Adjustment Today? Yes or No

Please describe how your body's old stress responses have changed. _____

_____

_____

Please describe what your daily goals are as your stress level improves.

_____

_____

_____

Time listened to AM02 Concentration _____ . Please rate your energy after listening.

No effect
1   2   3   4   5   6   7   8
                                    (8) I am energized and ready for the day

Which SMT Session did you listen to: _____

What action steps will you take after listening?

_____

_____

What changed in your ability to handle your daily stress?

_____

_____

Write any happy moments from the last 24 hours here?

_____

_____

List any activies here that prove your "energy" is improving?

_____

_____

List any victories over stress in your daily life?

_____

_____

Take a moment to list those things you are grateful for.

_____

_____

_____

List any compliments you received over the past 24 hours. Or, positive thoughts you have had about yourself or life.

_____

_____

_____

What type of exercise did you do today?

_____

_____

_____

What steps did you take today to improve the relationships in your life?

_____

_____

_____

Write one of your goals as if you have already accomplished it?

_____

_____

_____

Observations from your day:

_____

_____

_____

Listen to PM02 Release Negativity.

Day 18 Date: ___ / ___ / ____
Chiropractic Adjustment Today? Yes or No

How has your body's old stress changed?
Hasn't Changed
1   2   3   4   5   6   7   8
                                                        (8) Eliminated

How would you rate your current level of stress.

Severe
1   2   3   4   5   6   7   8
                                                        (8) Nonexistent

Time listened to AM03 Motivation _____ . Please rate your energy after listening.

No effect
1   2   3   4   5   6   7   8
                                        (8) I am energized and ready for the day

Which SMT Session did you listen to: _____
How would you rate your relaxation during the session.

I didn't relax at all
1   2   3   4   5   6   7   8
                                        (8) I can't image going deeper

How "confident" do you feel about your ability to handle your daily stress?

Not confident at all
1   2   3   4   5   6   7   8
                                                (8) Very confident

How "positive" is your attitude—in other words, how happy are you?

Very negative and unhappy
1   2   3   4   5   6   7   8
                                (8) Very positive—couldn't be happier!

How much "energy" do you have today?

No energy at all
1   2   3   4   5   6   7   8
                                        (8) All the energy I need

How well did you "sleep" last night?

Not well at all
1   2   3   4   5   6   7   8
                                        (8) Great—I'm well rested

How much "stress" do you feel about your daily life?

Very stressed all the time
1   2   3   4   5   6   7   8

(8) Stress-free: nothing bothers me

How would your rate your "overall health" outlook?

Many serious health concerns
1   2   3   4   5   6   7   8

(8) My doctor says I'm in great shape!

How much "self-esteem" do you have and how many "compliments" do you receive?

No self-esteem at all/
No one compliments me
1   2   3   4   5   6   7   8

(8) Very high self-esteem. I get tons of compliments

Do you feel you get enough "exercise"?

No exercise at all
1   2   3   4   5   6   7   8

(8) Exercise daily

How would you rate the significant "relationships" in your life?

Very unhappy/
No relationships in my life
1   2   3   4   5   6   7   8

(8) Extremely happy/
My relationships are the highlight of my life

How confident are you that you will reach your ultimate goal?

Not confident at all
1   2   3   4   5   6   7   8

(8) Very confident

If less than 4 above what stops you from being confident? _____

_____ _____

_____ _____

Observations from your day:

_____ _____

_____ _____

_____ _____

Listen to PM03 Creating Your Success Time-line

Day 19 Date: ___ / ___ / ____
Chiropractic Adjustment Today? Yes or No

1) Where in your body do you hold or carry your stress? _____

_____

_____

2) How would you rate your current level of stress?

Hasn't Changed
1   2   3   4   5   6   7   8
                                                (8) Eliminated

3) Time listened to AM01 Focus _____ . *Please rate your energy after listening.*

No effect
1   2   3   4   5   6   7   8
                          (8) I am energized and ready for the day

4) Which SMT Session did you listen to: _____

5) How would you rate your relaxation during the session.

I didn't relax at all
1   2   3   4   5   6   7   8
                                  (8) I can't imagine going deeper

6) How "confident" do you feel about your ability to handle your daily stress?

Not confident at all
1   2   3   4   5   6   7   8
                                                (8) Very confident

How "positive" is your attitude—in other words, how happy are you?

Very negative and unhappy
1   2   3   4   5   6   7   8
                          (8) Very positive—couldn't be happier!

7) How much "energy" do you have?

No energy at all
1   2   3   4   5   6   7   8
                                        (8) All the energy I want

8) How well do you "sleep"?

Not well at all
1   2   3   4   5   6   7   8
                                    (8) Great—I'm well rested

9) How much "stress" do you feel in your daily life?

Very stressed all the time
1   2   3   4   5   6   7   8

(8) Stress-free: nothing bothers me

10) How would your rate your "overall health"?

Many serious health concerns
1   2   3   4   5   6   7   8
(8) My doctor says I'm in great shape!

11) How much "self-esteem" do you have and how many "compliments" do you receive?

No self-esteem at all/
No one compliments me
1   2   3   4   5   6   7   8
(8) Very high self-esteem. I get tons of compliments

12) Do you feel you get enough "exercise"?

No exercise at all
1   2   3   4   5   6   7   8
(8) Exercise daily

13) How would you rate the significant "relationships" in your life?

Very unhappy/
No relationships in my life
1   2   3   4   5   6   7   8
(8) Extremely happy/
My relationships are the highlight of my life

14) How confident are you that you will reach your ultimate goal?

Not confident at all
1   2   3   4   5   6   7   8
(8) Very confident

15) If less than 4 above, what stops you from being confident?

_____

_____ _____

_____ _____

16) Observations from your day:

_____ _____

_____ _____

_____ _____

Day 20 Date: ___ / ___ / ____
Chiropractic Adjustment Today? Yes or No

Please describe how your body's old stress responses have changed. _____
_____
_____

Please describe what your daily goals are as your stress level improves.
_____
_____
_____

Time listened to AM02 Concentration _____ . *Please rate your energy after listening.*

No effect
1   2   3   4   5   6   7   8
(8) I am energized and ready for the day

Which SMT Session did you listen to: _____

What action steps will you take after listening?
_____
_____
_____

What changed in your ability to handle your daily stress?
_____
_____
_____

Write any happy moments from the last 24 hours here?
_____
_____
_____

List any activies here that prove your "energy" is improving?
_____
_____
_____

List any victories over stress in your daily life?
_____
_____

Take a moment to list those things you are grateful for.

_____

_____

_____

List any compliments you received over the past 24 hours. Or, positive thoughts you have had about yourself or life.

_____

_____

_____

What type of exercise did you do today?

_____

_____

_____

What steps did you take today to improve the relationships in your life?

_____

_____

_____

Write one of your goals as if you have already accomplished it?

_____

_____

_____

_____

Observations from your day:

_____

_____

_____

_____

Listen to PM02 Release Negativity.

Day 21 Date: ___ / ___ / ____
Chiropractic Adjustment Today? Yes or No

How has your body's old stress changed?
Hasn't Changed
1   2   3   4   5   6   7   8
                                        (8) Eliminated

How would you rate your current level of stress.

Severe
1   2   3   4   5   6   7   8
                                        (8) Nonexistent

Time listened to AM03 Motivation _____ . Please rate your energy after listening.

No effect
1   2   3   4   5   6   7   8
                            (8) I am energized and ready for the day.

Which SMT Session did you listen to: _____
How would you rate your relaxation during the session.

I didn't relax at all
1   2   3   4   5   6   7   8
                                (8) I can't image going deeper

How "confident" do you feel about your ability to handle your daily stress?

Not confident at all
1   2   3   4   5   6   7   8
                                        (8) Very confident

How "positive" is your attitude—in other words, how happy are you?

Very negative and unhappy
1   2   3   4   5   6   7   8
                        (8) Very positive—couldn't be happier!

How much "energy" do you have today?

No energy at all
1   2   3   4   5   6   7   8
                                (8) All the energy I need

How well did you "sleep" last night?

Not well at all
1   2   3   4   5   6   7   8
                                (8) Great—I'm well rested

How much "stress" do you feel about your daily life?

Very stressed all the time
1   2   3   4   5   6   7   8

(8) Stress-free: nothing bothers me

How would your rate your "overall health" outlook?

Many serious health concerns
1   2   3   4   5   6   7   8

(8) My doctor says I'm in great shape!

How much "self-esteem" do you have and how many "compliments" do you receive?

No self-esteem at all/
No one compliments me
1   2   3   4   5   6   7   8

(8) Very high self-esteem. I get tons of compliments

Do you feel you get enough "exercise"?

No exercise at all
1   2   3   4   5   6   7   8

(8) Exercise daily

How would you rate the significant "relationships" in your life?

Very unhappy/
No relationships in my life
1   2   3   4   5   6   7   8

(8) Extremely happy/
My relationships are the highlight of my life

How confident are you that you will reach your ultimate goal?

Not confident at all
1   2   3   4   5   6   7   8

(8) Very confident

If less than 4 above what stops you from being confident? _____

_____   _____

_____   _____

Observations from your day:

_____   _____

_____   _____

_____   _____

Listen to PM03 Creating Your Success Time-line

21-Day Tracking

Sample: Please collect your results from the "21 Day Tracker." Post them here and see your results.

Eliminated

Hasn't Changed

| Day One | Four | Seven | Ten | Thirteen | Sixteen | Nineteen |

Notes: *I feel less stress at work and I am now sleeping through the night.*

_____

_____

_____

_____

21-Day Tracking

Question #2
How would you rate your current level of stress?

Eliminated

8	8	8	8	8	8	8
7	7	7	7	7	7	7
6	6	6	6	6	6	6
5	5	5	5	5	5	5
4	4	4	4	4	4	4
3	3	3	3	3	3	3
2	2	2	2	2	2	2
1	1	1	1	1	1	1

Hasn't Changed

Day One	Four	Seven	Ten	Thirteen	Sixteen	Nineteen

Notes: _____

_____

_____

_____

_____

21-Day Tracking

3) Time listened to AM01 Focus.
Please rate your energy after listening.
(8) I am energized and ready for the day

8	8	8	8	8	8	8
7	7	7	7	7	7	7
6	6	6	6	6	6	6
5	5	5	5	5	5	5
4	4	4	4	4	4	4
3	3	3	3	3	3	3
2	2	2	2	2	2	2
1	1	1	1	1	1	1

No effect

Day One	Four	Seven	Ten	Thirteen	Sixteen	Nineteen

Notes: _____

_____

_____

_____

_____

21-Day Tracking

5) How would you rate your relaxation during the session.

(8) I can't imagine going deeper

8	8	8	8	8	8	8
7	7	7	7	7	7	7
6	6	6	6	6	6	6
5	5	5	5	5	5	5
4	4	4	4	4	4	4
3	3	3	3	3	3	3
2	2	2	2	2	2	2
1	1	1	1	1	1	1

I didn't relax at all

| Day One | Four | Seven | Ten | Thirteen | Sixteen | Nineteen |

Notes: _____

_____

_____

_____

_____

21-Day Tracking

6) How "confident" do you feel about your ability to handle your daily stress?

(8) Very confident

8	8	8	8	8	8	8
7	7	7	7	7	7	7
6	6	6	6	6	6	6
5	5	5	5	5	5	5
4	4	4	4	4	4	4
3	3	3	3	3	3	3
2	2	2	2	2	2	2
1	1	1	1	1	1	1

Not confident at all

| Day One | Four | Seven | Ten | Thirteen | Sixteen | Nineteen |

Notes: _____

_____

_____

_____

_____

21-Day Tracking

7) How "positive" is your attitude—in other words, how happy are you?

(8) Very positive—couldn't be happier!

	8	8	8	8	8	8	8
	7	7	7	7	7	7	7
	6	6	6	6	6	6	6
	5	5	5	5	5	5	5
	4	4	4	4	4	4	4
	3	3	3	3	3	3	3
	2	2	2	2	2	2	2
	1	1	1	1	1	1	1

Very negative and unhappy

Day One	Four	Seven	Ten	Thirteen	Sixteen	Nineteen

Notes: _____

_____

_____

_____

_____

21-Day Tracking

8) How much "energy" do you have?

(8) All the energy I want

8	8	8	8	8	8	8
7	7	7	7	7	7	7
6	6	6	6	6	6	6
5	5	5	5	5	5	5
4	4	4	4	4	4	4
3	3	3	3	3	3	3
2	2	2	2	2	2	2
1	1	1	1	1	1	1

No energy at all

Day One   Four   Seven   Ten   Thirteen   Sixteen   Nineteen

Notes: _____

_____

_____

_____

_____

21-Day Tracking

9) How well do you "sleep"?

(8) Great—I'm well rested

8	8	8	8	8	8	8
7	7	7	7	7	7	7
6	6	6	6	6	6	6
5	5	5	5	5	5	5
4	4	4	4	4	4	4
3	3	3	3	3	3	3
2	2	2	2	2	2	2
1	1	1	1	1	1	1

Not well at all

| Day One | Four | Seven | Ten | Thirteen | Sixteen | Nineteen |

Notes: _____

_____

_____

_____

_____

21-Day Tracking

10) How much "stress" do you feel in your daily life?

(8) Stress-free: nothing bothers me

8	8	8	8	8	8	8
7	7	7	7	7	7	7
6	6	6	6	6	6	6
5	5	5	5	5	5	5
4	4	4	4	4	4	4
3	3	3	3	3	3	3
2	2	2	2	2	2	2
1	1	1	1	1	1	1

Very stressed all the time

Day One	Four	Seven	Ten	Thirteen	Sixteen	Nineteen

Notes: _____

_____

_____

_____

_____

21-Day Tracking

11) How would your rate your "overall health"?

(8) My doctor says I'm in great shape!

8	8	8	8	8	8	8
7	7	7	7	7	7	7
6	6	6	6	6	6	6
5	5	5	5	5	5	5
4	4	4	4	4	4	4
3	3	3	3	3	3	3
2	2	2	2	2	2	2
1	1	1	1	1	1	1

Many serious health concerns

Day One	Four	Seven	Ten	Thirteen	Sixteen	Nineteen

Notes: _____

_____

_____

_____

_____

21-Day Tracking

12) How much "self-esteem" do you have and how many "compliments" do you receive?

(8) Very high self-esteem. I get tons of compliments

8	8	8	8	8	8	8
7	7	7	7	7	7	7
6	6	6	6	6	6	6
5	5	5	5	5	5	5
4	4	4	4	4	4	4
3	3	3	3	3	3	3
2	2	2	2	2	2	2
1	1	1	1	1	1	1

No self-esteem at all. No one compliments me

Day One	Four	Seven	Ten	Thirteen	Sixteen	Nineteen

Notes: _____

_____

_____

_____

_____

21-Day Tracking

13) Do you feel you get enough "exercise"?

No exercise at all

8	8	8	8	8	8	8
7	7	7	7	7	7	7
6	6	6	6	6	6	6
5	5	5	5	5	5	5
4	4	4	4	4	4	4
3	3	3	3	3	3	3
2	2	2	2	2	2	2
1	1	1	1	1	1	1

(8) Exercise daily

Day One   Four   Seven   Ten   Thirteen   Sixteen   Nineteen

Notes: _____

_____

_____

_____

_____

21-Day Tracking

14) How would you rate the significant "relationships" in your life?

Very unhappy/ No relationships in my life

8	8	8	8	8	8	8
7	7	7	7	7	7	7
6	6	6	6	6	6	6
5	5	5	5	5	5	5
4	4	4	4	4	4	4
3	3	3	3	3	3	3
2	2	2	2	2	2	2
1	1	1	1	1	1	1

(8) Extremely happy/ My relationships are the highlight of my life

| Day One | Four | Seven | Ten | Thirteen | Sixteen | Nineteen |

Notes: _____

_____

_____

_____

_____

21-Day Tracking

15) How confident are you that you will reach your ultimate goal?

(8) Very confident

8	8	8	8	8	8	8
7	7	7	7	7	7	7
6	6	6	6	6	6	6
5	5	5	5	5	5	5
4	4	4	4	4	4	4
3	3	3	3	3	3	3
2	2	2	2	2	2	2
1	1	1	1	1	1	1

Not confident at all

Day One	Four	Seven	Ten	Thirteen	Sixteen	Nineteen

Notes: _____

_____

_____

_____

_____

How many Chiropractic Adjustments did you receive during the 21 Day Action Plan? _____ What benefits did you notice? _____

_____   _____

_____   _____

What would you accomplish if you knew you couldn't fail?

_____   _____

_____   _____

_____   _____

_____   _____

What observations from the last 21 days will help you accomplish future goals?

_____   _____

_____   _____

_____   _____

_____   _____

_____   _____

_____   _____

List out your top ten goals:

1) _____

2) _____

3) _____

4) _____

5) _____

6) _____

7) _____

8) _____

9) _____

10) _____

CHAPTER
EIGHTEEN

ADDITIONAL

RESOURCES

Brain Based Wellness Books

1. Brain Rules by John Medina

2. Evolve the Brain by Joe Dispenza

3. A Symphony in the Brain by Jim Robbins

4. The Reality Check by Heidi Haavik

5. Spark by John Ratay

6. Why You Get Sick and How Your Brain Can Fix It by

   Richard Barwell

7. Autism by Robert Melillo

8. Holographic Healing by George Gonzalez

9. The Brain that Changes Itself by Norman Doidge

10. Mind over Medicine by Lissa Rankin

11. Thrive In Overdrive, How to navigate Your Overload-

    ed Lifestyle by Patrick K. Porter, Ph.D.

Awaken the Genius, Mind Technology for the 21st

   Century by Patrick K. Porter, Ph.D.

Dr. Patrick Porter's
Stress-Free Lifestyle Series

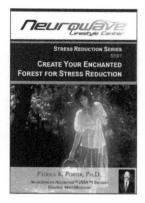

Stress is the most pervasive malady of our time. The effects on our health, productivity and quality of life are more devastating than most people care to admit. Luckily, you've just found the solution! CVR can help you see yourself as the healthy, happy, optimistic person you'd prefer to be. With this new image, your fears and frustrations fade away, your anxiety vanishes, and you no longer let small things stress you.

Vibrant Health Series

Of all the cells in your body, more than 50,000 will die and be replaced with new cells, all in the time it took you to read this sentence! Your body is the vehicle you have been given for the journey of your life. How you treat your body determines how it will treat you. Taking good care of your body will go a long way in ensuring that your life is active, happy, and full of positive experiences. Dr. Patrick Porter will show you how, by using creative visualization and relaxation (CVR), you can recharge and energize your body, mind, and spirit. This series is for people who are looking for more than good health; it's for those who will settle for nothing less than vibrant health!

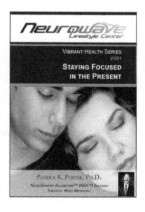

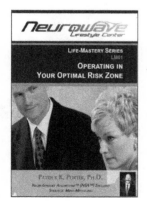

Life-Mastery Series

Throughout your life, from parents, teachers, and society, you were taught what to think. With the breakthrough processes of creative visualization and relaxation, you are going to discover how to think. With this knowledge you will literally become a software engineer for your own mind. On the Life-Mastery journey, you will explore the processes that best suit your needs for creating limitless personal improvement and success in your life.

at **http://smtstreaming.com/crt**

Wealth Consciousness Series

Inspired by the principles of Napoleon Hill's
Think and Grow Rich

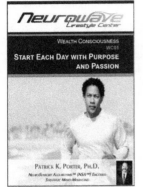

Start Each Day with Purpose and Passion
Napoleon Hill understood that people don't plan to fail; they fail to plan. Successful people know where they are going before they start and move forward on their own initiative. They have the power of intention, or what Napoleon Hill called "mind energy," on their side. Dr. Patrick Porter (PhD) will guide you in using this power of intention to focus your imagination on the success and prosperity you desire.

Weight Control Series

Now you can design the body you want and the life you love. That's right, you can have the trim, healthy body you've always dreamed of by simply changing the way you see yourself and your life. Once you have a new image of yourself, everything else changes—junk food and fast food lose their appeal, healthy foods become desirable, and you eat only when you're hungry. With Dr. Porter's System you will overcome common weight loss mistakes, learn to eat and think like a naturally thin person, conquer cravings, and increase your self-confidence. Each week you will take another step toward a lifetime of healthy living; losing weight is the natural byproduct of these changes. While the average diet lasts just 72 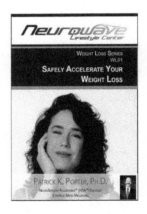 hours and focuses on depriving you of the foods you love, Dr. Patrick Porter supercharges your weight loss motivation with these powerful creative visualization and relaxation processes! You will eliminate the problem where it started— your own mind. There is simply no easier way to lose weight than CVR!

at **http://smtstreaming.com/crt**

Accelerated Learning Series

Whether you are an honor student or just having difficulty taking a test, this breakthrough learning system will help you overcome learning challenges and accelerate your current skill level. Imagine doubling your reading speed while improving your memory. Sit back, relax and allow your mind to organize your life, while you build your self-confidence and earn better grades with the our complete learning system.

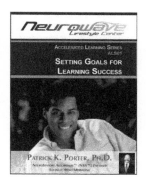

Freedom From Addiction Series

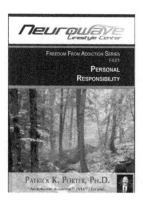

Addiction comes in many forms, but the underlying cause remains the same. For every addiction there is an underlying positive intention that the mind is trying to fulfill. Now you can use the power of your mind—through creative visualization and relaxation (CVR)—to find more appropriate ways to satisfy that positive intention without the destructive behaviors of the past. Dr. Patrick Porter's groundbreaking CVR program for overcoming addiction can work for just about any addiction including the following: *Alcoholism, Anorexia & Bulimia, Codependency, Gambling, Marijuana, Narcotics.*

Coping with Cancer Series

Being diagnosed with cancer is in itself a stressful event—so stressful it can suppress your immune system and worsen the side-effects of treatment. Fortunately, through guided relaxation, you can let go of your fear and anxiety, and take charge of your recovery. Creative visualization can help you regain an optimistic attitude, spark your immune system, and maximize your medical treatment. If you are ready to join the ranks of people who have discovered the mind/body connection and its healing potential, then the Coping with Cancer Series is definitely for you!

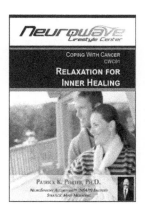

at http://smtstreaming.com/crt

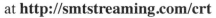

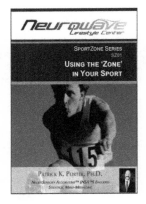

SportZone™ Series

Success in sports is about being the best you can be, and visualization plays a key role in getting there. Why is visualization so important? Because you get what you rehearse in life, but that's not always what you want or intend. This is especially true when you are facing the pressures of athletics. The SportZone program is designed to help you tap into the mind's potential and make your sport of choice fun and enjoyable while taking your game to the next level. Visualization for sports performance is nothing new to top competitors—athletes from Tiger Woods to diver Greg Louganis and a variety of Olympians have used visualization to bring about optimal performance, overcome self-doubt, and give themselves a seemingly unfair advantage over their competition. Now the SportZone series can work for any athlete, from junior competitors to weekend enthusiasts. Yes, you can get more out of your sport and, in the process, get more out of life.

Smoking Cessation Series

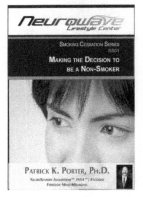

Kicking your smoking habit doesn't get any easier or more fun than this! When you use Dr. Patrick Porter's proven strategies, you'll find that making this life-saving change comes about simply and effortlessly. With the new science of creative visualization and relaxation (CVR), you will extinguish the stress and frustration associated with quitting smoking, and you'll conquer your cravings like the tens of thousands of others who have used Dr. Porter's processes.

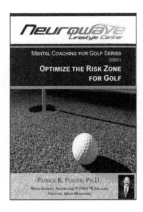

Mental Coaching for Golf Series

Efficient golfers know how to relax and let their minds take over. Now, thanks to these creative visualization and relaxation (CVR) processes, you'll learn to see yourself as a calm, confident golfer. You deserve to take pleasure in your time on the course. Thanks to CVR, you'll finally be able to let go of frustration and focus on every stroke—meaning you'll not only play better, but you'll also enjoy the game more than ever!

at **http://smtstreaming.com/crt**

Enlightened Children's Series

Seven-year-old Marina Mulac and five-year-old Morgan Mulac, who have come to be known as the world's youngest marketers, were the inspiration behind this Enlightened Children's Series. When they met Dr. Patrick Porter, they had one question for him: Why had he created so many great visualizations for grown ups and nothing for kids?

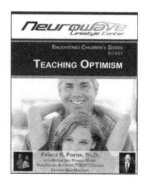

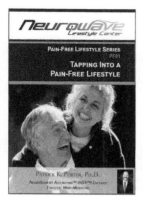

Pain-Free Lifestyle Series

Persistent pain can have a costly impact on your life. It can lead to depression, loss of appetite, irritability, anger, loss of sleep, withdrawal from social interaction, and an inability to cope. Fortunately, with creative visualization and relaxation (CVR), pain can almost always be controlled. CVR helps you eliminate pain while you relax, revitalize, and rejuvenate. You deserve to be free of your pain—and now you can be, thanks to CVR!

Stress-Free Childbirth Series

Bringing a child into the world should be an amazing life experience. Sadly, for many women, the joy of the event is lost due to fear, stress and pain. Also, research has shown that a fetus can actually feel the stress, worry, and negative emotions of the mother during pregnancy. Fortunately, with the discovery of the mind/body connection, women have an alternative—creative visualization and relaxation (CVR). This breakthrough series is designed to help the mother-to-be to relax, let go of stress, and enjoy the entire process of pregnancy, delivery and motherhood. In addition, the listener is taught to use the power of thought to create an anaesthetized feeling that can transform pain into pressure throughout labor and delivery—making the entire process stress-free for the entire family.

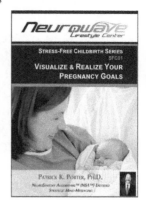

at **http://smtstreaming.com/crt**

The Way Back to Health

There IS a way back to balanced, stress-free health and well-being. It's called the Cranial Release Technique®. Research shows that the Cranial Release Process causes the brain to come out of the "stress-state" and to return back to balanced function again. This not only helps to balance the body structure, but also creates balance within body physiology leading to proper organ function and healing. All of this can put you back on the path to true, high-level health and wellness.

Are You Stressed?

Here's the good news: Your Cranial Release Practitioner can screen you to see if stress is having a negative impact on your well-being. It's fast, fun and highly informative. If signs of stress are present, they'll give you more information on how Cranial Release Technique® can help you.

The Benefits of CRT:
- Balanced Body Structure/Muscles
- Greater Mind Focus and Calmness
- Relief of Pain in Neck and Back
- Better Sleep • More Energy
- Improved Outlook on Life
- Enhanced Creativity
- Ability to better handle stress and life
- Lightness, Clarity, less negativity
- Headaches disappear
- Improved Strength and Performance

Do You Suffer From:
- Pain in the Neck or Back
- Difficulty Sleeping
- Short Term Memory Loss
- Difficulty Focusing
- Headaches/Migraines
- Adrenal Fatigue/Exhaustion
- Negative Self-talk/Anxiety

Do you realize that all these symptoms and more can be caused by stress? 90% of all illness can be linked to stress.

The Way Back To Health

There's no question that we live in stressful times, and our stress levels are increasing every year. Scientists have actually coined the term "Complex Stress" to describe today's fast paced, always on the go lifestyle. Nearly every moment of every day we're confronted with one type of stress or another. From multi-tasking on the job, to ferrying the kids to after school activities, to the constant stream of e-mails, cell phone calls, text messages, and it goes on and on. While all these stressful events are certainly not life-threatening, our body's reaction to them is the same as if they are, and that can have devastating effects on our health and well-being.

Stress and the Brain

It is now recognized that chronic stress has significant negative effects on the brain and central nervous system. Our chronic stress can cause the brain to "lock" into an almost permanent "fight or flight" state. This results in one brain hemisphere becoming overly active or dominant and the other in effect shutting down and reducing in activity.

Structure

This "stress state" in the brain creates imbalance within the muscular system of the body leading to abnormal stress on the spine and joints. This structural imbalance can lead to injury, pain, weakness, poor performance and degeneration.

Function

The long term "fight or flight" state also leads to imbalance of the autonomic nervous system, with the sympathetic or "fight or flight" system becoming predominant. This often leads to problems with day to day activities such as indigestion, ulcers, poor bowel habits, sleep disturbances, blood sugar problems, poor immune system function, high blood pressure, fatigue, slow healing and repair. This happens because the Life Energy of the body perceives our constant stress as a threat to survival, it then places it's focus on defending us rather than on the healing and regeneration of body tissues and organs. Chronic illness, pain and poor health is the inevitable result.

For More Information
Call 917-400-1911
http://theultimatewellnesspractice.com

Welcome to The Gift of Love Project

The Gift of Love is a poetic writing that has its own beauty … and upon further examination, it may lead one to a contemplative process, creating balance and harmony in one's everyday life. Over time, this process can also create subtle positive change in the recipient of **The Gift**.

My guidance leads me to distribute this writing to one billion people within the next two years. Hopefully, many people will be led to practice the contemplative process. If **The Gift of Love** resonates with you, please share it with others. As we gather and hold the **power of love** in our consciousness, we will dramatically reduce the level of anger, fear, and hatred on our planet today. -- Jerry DeShazo

The Gift of Love

I Agree Today
To Be The Gift of Love.

I Agree to Feel Deeply
Love for Others
Independent of Anything
They Are Expressing,
Saying, Doing, or Being.

I Agree to Allow Love
As I Know It
To Embrace My Whole Body
And Then to Just Send It
To Them Silently and Secretly.

I Agree to Feel it, Accept it, Breathe It
Into Every Cell of My Body on Each In-Breath
And On Each Out-Breath
Exhale Any Feeling Unlike Love.

I Will Repeat This Breathing Process Multiple Times
Until I Feel it Fully and Completely
Then Consciously Amplify In Me
The Feeling of Love and Project It to Others
As The Gift of Love.

This is My Secret Agreement –
No One Else Is To Know it.

For more about The Gift of Love Project and to view the videos, please visit www.TheGiftofLove.com. You will also be given access to a special 9-minute Creative Visualization that will align you with the **Power of Love** and supercharge your day. Together we will change the world one person at a time.

CPSIA information can be obtained
at www.ICGtesting.com
Printed in the USA
BVHW080737140620
581357BV00002B/64

9 781937 111298